The Exhaustive Sirtfood Diet (

Burn fat and Stay healthy effectively Activating Your Skinny Gene. 500 Fast, Simple and Tasty Recipes Cookbook + Easy 4 weeks Weight Loss Program

Anne Patel

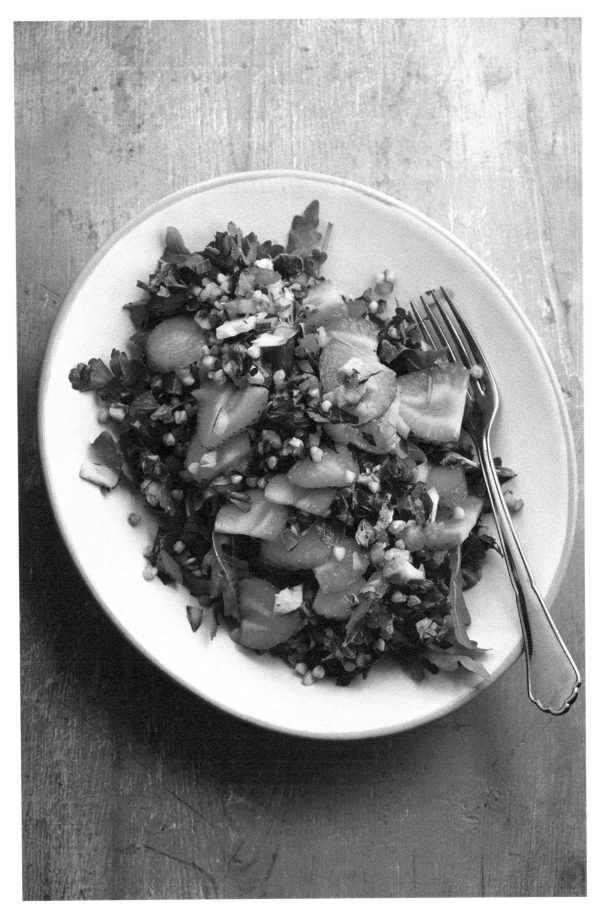

Table of contents

Breakfast

1. Sirt Muesli

Preparation time: 10 minutes - Cooking time: 0 minutes - Serves: 1

- 0.9-ounce buckwheat flakes
- 0.45 ounce of buckwheat puffs
- 1 ounce of Medjool dates, pitted and chopped Walnuts, chopped
- Coconut flakes or desiccated coconut
- 3.5 ounce of strawberries, hulled and chopped
- 0.45 ounce of cocoa nibs
- 3.5 ounce of plain Greek yogurt

1. You need to mix the dry ingredients and place them in an airtight container if you want to make it in a large amount or prepare it the night before.

Nutrition: Calories: 104, Sodium: 33 mg, Dietary Fiber: 1.4 g, Total Fat: 4.1 g, Total Carbs: 16.3 g, Protein: 1.3 g.

2. Lamb, Butternut Squash and Date Tagine

Preparation Time: 15 minutes - Cooking time: 40 minutes - Servings: 4 to 6

- 2 tablespoons olive oil
- 2cm ginger, grated
- 1 red onion, sliced
- 3 garlic cloves, grated or crushed
- 1 teaspoon chili flake (or to taste)
- 1 cinnamon stick
- 2 teaspoons cumin seeds
- 2 teaspoons ground turmeric
- ½ teaspoon salt
- Lamb neck fillet, cut into 2cm chunks
- Medjool dates, pitted and chopped
- 14 ounces of tin chopped tomatoes, plus half a can of water
- 14 ounces of tin chickpeas, drained
- 15.5 ounces of butternut squash, cut into 1cm cubes
- 2 tablespoons fresh coriander (plus extra for garnish)
- Buckwheat, couscous, flatbreads or rice to serve

1. Preheat the oven until 140C.

2. Sprinkle about two tablespoons of olive oil in a large oven-proof casserole dish or cast-iron pot. Put the sliced onion and cook on a gentle heat until the onions softened but not brown, with the lid on for about 5 minutes.

3. Add chili, cumin, cinnamon and turmeric to the grated garlic and ginger. Remove well, and cook the lid off for one more minute. If it gets too dry, add a drop of water.

4. Add pieces of lamb. In the onions and spices, stir well to coat the meat and then add salt, chopped dates and tomatoes, plus about half a can of water (100- 200ml).

5. Bring the tagine to the boil, then put the lid on and put it for 1 hour and 15 minutes in your preheated oven.

6. Add the chopped butternut squash and drained chickpeas thirty minutes before the end of the cooking time. Stir all together, bring the lid back on and go back to the oven for the remaining 30 minutes of cooking.

7. Remove from the oven when the tagine is finished, and stir through the chopped coriander. Serve with couscous, buckwheat, flatbreads, or basmati rice.

Notes:

If you don't own an oven-proof casserole dish or cast-iron casserole, cook the tagine in a regular casserole until it has to go into the oven and then transfer the tagine to a regular lidded casserole dish before placing it in the oven. Add 5 minutes of cooking time to provide enough time to heat the casserole dish.

Nutrition: Calories: 104, Sodium: 33 mg, Dietary Fiber: 1.4 g, Total Fat: 4.1 g, Total Carbs: 16.3 g, Protein: 1.3 g.

3. Chicken With Kale, Red Onions and Chili Salsa

Preparation time: 5 Minutes - Cooking Time: 70 Minutes - Servings: 2

For the salsa:

- 130g tomatoes
- 1 Thai chilies, finely chopped
- 1 tablespoon capers, finely chopped
- 5 g parsley, finely chopped
- Juice of a quarter of a lemon

For the rest:

- 3 ounces of chicken breast
- 2 teaspoons turmeric
- Juice of a quarter of a lemon
- 1 tablespoon of olive oil
- 1 ounce of kale, chopped
- 1 ounce of red onions, sliced
- 1 teaspoon chopped ginger
- 1.5 ounces of buckwheat

1. It is best to prepare the salsa first: remove the stalk of the tomato, chop it finely and mix it well with the other ingredients.

2. Preheat the oven to 425 °. In the meantime, marinate the chicken breast in some olive oil and a teaspoon of turmeric.

3. Heat an ovenproof pan on the stove and sauté the marinated chicken for one minute on each side. Then bake, remove and cover with aluminum foil in the oven for around 10 minutes.

4. In the meantime, briefly steam the kale. In a small saucepan, heat the red onions and ginger with olive oil until they become translucent, then add the kale and heat again.

5. Prepare buckwheat according to package Directions, serve with meat and vegetables.

Nutrition: Calories: 104, Sodium: 33 mg, Dietary Fiber: 1.4 g, Total Fat: 4.1 g, Total Carbs: 16.3 g, Protein: 1.3 g.

4. Tofu With Cauliflower

Preparation time: 5 Minutes - Cooking time: 45 Minutes - Servings 2

- 2 ounces of red pepper, seeded
- 1 Thai chilies, cut in two halves, seeded
- 2 cloves of garlic
- 1 teaspoon of olive oil
- 1 pinch of cumin
- 1 pinch of coriander
- Juice of a 1/4 lemon
- 7 ounces of tofu
- 7 ounces of cauliflower, roughly chopped
- 1 ounce of red onions, finely chopped
- 1 teaspoon finely chopped ginger
- 2 teaspoons turmeric
- 2-ounce dried tomatoes, finely chopped
- 2 ounces of parsley, chopped

1. Preheat oven to 400 °. Slice the peppers and put them in an ovenproof dish with chili and garlic. Pour some olive oil over it, add the dried herbs, put it in the oven for about 20 minutes, until the peppers are tender. Let it cool down, put the peppers together with the lemon juice in a blender and work it into a soft mass.

2. Cut the tofu in half and divide the halves into triangles. Place the tofu in a small casserole dish, cover with the paprika mixture and place in the oven for about 20 minutes.

3. Chop the cauliflower until the pieces are smaller than a grain of rice.

4. Then, in a small saucepan, heat the garlic, onions, chili and ginger with olive oil until they become transparent. Add turmeric and cauliflower, mix well and heat again. Remove from heat and add parsley and tomatoes, mix well. Serve with the tofu in the sauce.

Nutrition: Calories: 304, Sodium: 73 mg, Dietary Fiber: 1.4 g, Total Fat: 4.1 g, Total Carbs: 1.3 g, Protein: 0.3 g.

5. *Horseradish Flaked Salmon Fillet & Kale*

Preparation time: 10 minutes - Cooking time: 30 minutes - Servings: 1

- 7oz of skinless, boneless salmon fillet
- 1.5oz of green beans
- 1.7oz of kale
- 1 tablespoon extra-virgin olive oil
- ½ garlic clove, crushed
- 1.4oz red onion, chopped
- 1 tablespoon fresh chives, chopped
- 1 tablespoon freshly chopped flat-leaf parsley
- 1 tablespoon low fat *crème fraiche*
- 1tablespoon horseradish sauce
- Juice of ¼ lemon
- A pinch of salt and pepper

1. Preheat the grill.

2. Sprinkle a salmon fillet with salt and pepper. Place under the grill for 10-15 minutes. Flake and set aside.

3. Using a steamer, cook the kale and green beans for 10 minutes.

4. In a skillet, warm the oil over a high heat. Add garlic and red onion and fry for 2-3 minutes. Toss in the kale and beans, and then cook for 1-2 minutes more.

5. Mix the chives, parsley, *crème fraiche*, horseradish, lemon juice, and flaked salmon.

6. Serve the kale and beans topped with the dressed flaked salmon.

Nutrition: Calories: 304, Sodium: 73 mg, Dietary Fiber: 1.4 g, Total Fat: 4.1 g, Total Carbs: 1.3 g, Protein: 0.3 g.

6. *Indulgent Yogurt*

Preparation Time: 10 minutes - Cooking Time: 0 minutes - Servings: 1

- 125 mixed berries
- 3.5oz of Greek yogurt
- 25 walnuts, chopped
- 0.9oz of dark chocolate (at least 85% cocoa solids), grated

1. Toss the mixed berries into a serving bowl. Cover with yogurt and top with chocolate and walnuts. Voila!

Nutrition: Calories:115 Carbs: 4g Fat: 8g Protein: 6g

7. *Frozen Gazpacho*

Preparation time: 10 minutes - Cooking time: 0 minutes - Servings: 2

- 2 large or 6 small tomatoes, chopped
- 1 avocado, seeded, sliced and picked (wait until prompted)
- 1 medium cucumber, chopped
- 1 small red onion, chopped
- 1 cup very finely chopped arugula
- ½ celery stalk, finely chopped
- 1 garlic clove, chopped or pressed
- ½ chili or a pinch of cayenne pepper
- 1 teaspoon of lime juice pinch of sea salt A pinch of pepper

1. Put the ingredients in a blender or food processor and let them beat gently. You don't want to mix too well, or you make a liquid instead of a soup. The gazpacho must be thick. After mixing, put in the refrigerator for about 1 hour. You can also leave it overnight.

2. Cut and remove the avocado just before eating. Serve half of the gazpacho in a cold bowl. Add the avocado slices and serve immediately.

Nutrition: Calories: 304, Sodium: 73 mg, Dietary Fiber: 1.4 g, Total Fat: 4.1 g, Total Carbs: 1.3 g, Protein: 0.3 g.

8. *Tomato Frittata*

Preparation time: 10 minutes - Cooking time: 20 minutes - Servings: 2

- 1.3oz cheddar cheese, grated
- 1.4oz kalamata olives, pitted and halved
- 8 cherry tomatoes, halved
- 4 large eggs
- 1 tablespoon fresh parsley, chopped
- 1 tablespoon fresh basil, chopped
- 1 tablespoon olive oil

1. Whisk the eggs together in a large mixing bowl. Toss in the parsley, basil, olives, tomatoes and cheese, stirring thoroughly.

2. Heat the olive oil in a small skillet over high heat. Pour in the frittata mixture and cook for 5-10 minutes, or set.

3. Remove the skillet from the hob and position for 5 minutes under the grill, or until firm and set. Divide into portions and serve immediately.

Nutrition: Calories: 304 Sodium: 73 mg Dietary Fiber: 1.4 g Total Fat: 4.1 g Total Carbs: 1.3 Protein: 0.3 g

9. *Chicken With Kale and Chili Salsa*

Preparation time: 5 Minutes - Cooking Time: 45 Minutes - Servings 1

- 3 ounces of buckwheat
- 1 teaspoon of chopped fresh ginger
- Juice of ½ lemon, divided
- 2 teaspoons of ground turmeric
- 3 ounces of kale, chopped
- 1.3 ounces of red onion, sliced
- 4 ounces of skinless, boneless chicken breast
- 1 tablespoon of extra-virgin olive oil
- 1 tomato
- 1 handful parsley
- 1 bird's eye chili, chopped

1. Start with the salsa: Remove the eye out of the tomato and finely chop it, make sure that you hold as much of the liquid

as possible. Mix it with the chili, parsley, and lemon juice. You could add everything to a blender for different results.

2. Heat your oven to 220 degrees F. Marinate the chicken with a little oil, 1 teaspoon of turmeric, and the lemon juice. Let it rest for 5-10 minutes.

3. Heat a pan until it is hot, over medium heat, then add marinated chicken and allow it to cook for a minute on both sides until it is pale gold). If the pan is not ovenproof, Put the chicken in the oven and bake in a baking dish for 8 to 10 minutes or until it is cooked through. Take the chicken out of the oven, cover it with foil, and let it stand before serving for five minutes.

4. Meanwhile, in a steamer, steam the kale for about 5 minutes.

5. In a little oil, fry the ginger and red onions until they are soft but not colored, and then add in the cooked kale and fry it for a minute.

6. Cook the buckwheat in accordance with the packet Directions with the remaining turmeric. Serve alongside the vegetables, salsa and chicken.

Nutrition: Calories: 304 Sodium: 73 mg Dietary Fiber: 1.4 g Total Fat: 4.1 g Total Carbs: 1.3 g Protein: 0.3 g

10. *Buckwheat Tuna Casserole*

Preparation time: 10 minutes - Cooking time: 35 minutes - Servings: 2
- 2 tablespoons butter
- 10-ounce package buckwheat ramen noodles
- 2 cups boiling water
- 1/3 cup dry red wine
- 3 cups milk
- 2 tablespoons dried parsley
- 2 teaspoons turmeric
- ½ teaspoon curry powder
- 2 tablespoons All-Purpose flour
- 2 cups celery, chopped
- 1 cup frozen peas
- 2 cans tuna, drained

1. Dot butter into your crockpot and grease the pot.

2. Place buckwheat ramen noodles in a large bowl and pour boiling water to cover. Let sit for 5 – 8 minutes, or until noodles separate when prodded with a fork.

3. Whisk the red wine together in a separate cup, milk, parsley, turmeric and flour.

4. Fold in celery, peas, and tuna.

5. Drain the ramen and place into crockpot, pouring the tuna mixture over the top. Mix to combine.

6. Cover and cook for 7 to 9 hours or less, stirring occasionally.

Nutrition: Calories: 304 Sodium: 73 mg Dietary Fiber: 1.4 g Total Fat: 4.1 g Total Carbs: 1.3 g Protein: 0.3 g

11. *Cheesy Crockpot Chicken and Vegetables*

Preparation time: 10 minutes - Cooking time: 45 minutes - Servings: 2
- 1/3 cup ham, diced
- 3 carrots, chopped
- 3 stalks celery, chopped
- 1 small yellow onion, diced
- 2 cups mushrooms, sliced
- 1 cup green beans, chopped
- ¼ cup water

- 4 boneless, skinless chicken breasts, cubed
- 1 cup chicken broth
- 1 cup milk
- 1 tablespoon parsley, chopped
- ¾ teaspoon poultry seasoning
- 1 tablespoon All-Purpose flour
- 1 cup cheddar cheese, shredded
- ¼ cup Parmesan, shredded

1. In a large bowl, combine ham, carrots, celery, onion, mushrooms, and green beans. Mix and transfer to your crockpot.

2. Layer the chicken on top, without mixing.

3. In the bowl, now empty, whisk broth, milk, parsley, poultry seasoning and flour together until well combined.

4. Fold in the cheddar and Parmesan.

5. Pour the mixture over the chicken. DO NOT STIR.

6. Cover and cook for 3-4 hours, or 6-8 hours at low temperatures.

Nutrition: Calories: 314 Sodium: 73 mg Dietary Fiber: 2.4 g Total Fat: 5.1 g Total Carbs: 1.3g Protein: 5.3 g

12. *Artichoke, Chicken and Capers*

Preparation time: 10 minutes - Cooking time: 55 minutes - Servings: 2
- 6 boneless, skinless chicken breasts
- 2 cups mushrooms, sliced
- 1 (14 ½ ounces) can diced tomatoes
- 1 (8 or 9 ounces) package frozen artichokes
- 1 cup chicken broth
- ¼ cup dry white wine
- 1 medium yellow onion, diced
- ½ cup Kalamata olives, sliced
- ¼ cup capers, drained
- 3 tablespoons chia seeds
- 3 teaspoons curry powder
- 1 teaspoon turmeric
- 3/4 teaspoon dried lovage
- Salt and pepper to taste
- 3 cups hot cooked buckwheat

1. Rinse chicken & set aside.

2. In a large bowl, combine mushrooms, tomatoes – with juice, frozen artichoke hearts, chicken broth, white wine, onion, olives and capers.

3. Stir in chia seeds, curry powder, turmeric, lovage, salt and pepper.

4. Pour half the mixture into your crockpot, add the chicken, and pour the remainder of the sauce over the top.

5. Cover and bake for 7 to 8 hours on low or 3 1/2 to 4 hours on high.

6. Serve with hot cooked buckwheat.

Nutrition: Calories: 314, Sodium: 73 mg, Dietary Fiber: 2.4 g, Total Fat: 5.1 g, Total Carbs: 1.3 g, Protein: 5.3 g.

13. *Chicken Merlot With Mushrooms*

Preparation time: 10 minutes - Cooking time: 40 minutes - Servings: 2
- 6 boneless, skinless chicken breasts, cubed
- 3 cups mushrooms, sliced
- 1 large red onion, chopped
- 2 cloves garlic, minced
- ¾ cup chicken broth
- 1 (6 ounces) can tomato paste
- ¼ cup Merlot

- 3 tablespoons chia seeds
- 2 tablespoons basil, chopped finely
- 2 teaspoons sugar
- Salt and pepper to taste
- 1 (10 ounces) package buckwheat ramen noodles, cooked
- 2 tablespoons Parmesan, shaved

1. Rinse chicken; set aside.
2. Add mushrooms, onion, and garlic to the crockpot and mix.
3. Place chicken cubes on top of the vegetables and do not mix.
4. Combine the broth and tomato paste in a large tub, wine, chia seeds, basil, sugar, salt, and pepper. Pour over the chicken.
5. Cover and cook on low for 7 to 8 hours or on high for 3 ½ to 4 hours.
6. Spoon chicken, mushroom mixture, and sauce over hot cooked ramen buckwheat noodles for serving. Top with shaved Parmesan.

Nutrition: Calories: 314, Sodium: 73 mg, Dietary Fiber: 2.4 g, Total Fat: 5.1 g, Total Carbs: 1.3 g, Protein: 5.3 g.

14. *Country Chicken Breasts*

Preparation time: 10 minutes - Cooking time: 45 minutes - Servings: 2

- 2 medium green apples, diced
- 1 small red onion, finely diced
- 1 small green bell pepper, chopped
- 3 cloves garlic, minced
- 2 tablespoons dried currants
- 1 tablespoon curry powder
- 1 teaspoon turmeric
- 1 teaspoon ground ginger
- ¼ teaspoon chili pepper flakes
- 1 can (14 ½ ounce) diced tomatoes
- 6 skinless, boneless chicken breasts, halved ½ cup chicken broth
- 1 cup long-grain white rice
- 1-pound large raw shrimp, shelled and deveined
- Salt and pepper to taste
- Chopped parsley
- 1/3 cup slivered almonds

1. Rinse chicken, pat dry, and set aside.
2. In a large crockpot, combine apples, onion, bell pepper, garlic, currants, curry powder, turmeric, ginger, and chili pepper flakes. Stir in tomatoes.
3. Arrange chicken, overlapping pieces slightly, on top of tomato mixture.
4. Pour in broth and do not mix or stir.
5. Cover and cook at about 6 – 7 hours on low.
6. Preheat oven to 200 degrees F.
7. Carefully transfer chicken to an oven-safe plate, cover lightly, and keep warm in the oven.
8. Stir the rice into the liquid that remains. Increase the heat to high in the cooker; cover and cook for 30 to 35 minutes, stir until the rice is almost tender to bite, once or twice. Stir in the shrimp, cover and cook for about 10 more minutes until the shrimp is opaque in the middle.
9. Meanwhile, toast almonds in a small pan over medium heat until golden brown, 5 - 8 minutes, stirring occasionally. Set aside.

10. To serve, season rice mixture to taste with salt and pepper. Mound in a warm serving dish and arrange chicken on top. Sprinkle with parsley and almonds.

Nutrition: Calories: 314, Sodium: 73 mg, Dietary Fiber: 2.4 g, Total Fat: 5.1 g, Total Carbs: 1.3 g, Protein: 5.3 g.

15. *Tuna and Kale*

Preparation time: 5 minutes - Cooking time: 20 minutes - Servings: 4

- 1-pound tuna fillets, boneless, skinless and cubed
- 2 tablespoons olive oil
- 1 cup kale, torn
- ½ cup cherry tomatoes, cubed
- 1 yellow onion, chopped

1. Over medium heat, heat the pan with the oil, add the onion and sauté for 5 minutes.
2. Add the tuna and the other ingredients, toss, cook everything for 15 minutes more, divide between plates and serve.

Nutrition: Calories: 314, Sodium: 73 mg, Dietary Fiber: 2.4 g, Total Fat: 5.1 g, Total Carbs: 1.3 g, Protein: 5.3 g.

16. *Turkey With Cauliflower Couscous*

Preparation time: 20 minutes - Cooking time: 50 minutes - Servings: 1

- 3 ounces of turkey
- 2-ounce g of cauliflower
- 2 ounces of red onion
- 1 teaspoon fresh ginger
- 1 pepper Bird's Eye
- 1 clove of garlic
- 3 tablespoons of extra virgin olive oil
- 2 teaspoons of turmeric
- 1.3 ounces of dried tomatoes
- 0.30ounces parsley
- Dried sage to taste
- 1 tablespoon of capers
- 1/4 of fresh lemon juice

1. Blend the raw cauliflower tops and cook them in a teaspoon of extra virgin olive oil, garlic, red onion, chili pepper, ginger, and a teaspoon of turmeric.
2. Leave to flavor on the fire for a minute, then add the chopped sun-dried tomatoes and 5 g of parsley. Season the turkey slice with a teaspoon of extra virgin olive oil, the dried sage and cook it in another teaspoon of extra virgin olive oil. Once ready, season with a tablespoon of capers, 1/4 of lemon juice, 5 g of parsley, a tablespoon of water and add the cauliflower.

Nutrition: Calories: 114, Sodium: 7.3 mg, Dietary Fiber: 2.4 g, Total Fat: 2.1 g, Total Carbs: 1.3 g, Protein: 5.3 g.

17. *Oriental Prawns With Buckwheat*

Preparation time: 20 minutes - Cooking time: 20 minutes - Servings: 1

- 3 ounces of shrimps
- 1 spoon of turmeric
- 1 spoon of extra-virgin oil
- 1.3 ounces of grain spaghetti
- Cooking water
- Salt
- 1 clove of garlic
- Bird's Eye chili
- 1 spoon of ginger

- Red onion
- 3 ounces of celery
- 1.3 ounces of green beans
- 1.7 ounces of kale
- Broth

1. Cook for 2-3 minutes the peeled prawns with 1 teaspoon of turmeric and 1 teaspoon of extra virgin olive oil. Boil the buckwheat noodles in salt-free water, drain and set aside.

2. Fry with another teaspoon of extra virgin olive oil, 1 clove of garlic, 1 Bird's Eye chili and 1 teaspoon of finely chopped fresh ginger, 20 g of red onion and 40 g of sliced celery, 75 g of chopped green beans, 50 g of curly kale roughly chopped.

3. Add 100 ml of broth and bring to a boil, letting it simmer until the vegetables are cooked and soft. Add the prawns, spaghetti, and 5 g of celery leaves, bring to the boil, and serve.

Nutrition: Calories: 114, Sodium: 7.3 mg, Dietary Fiber: 2.4 g, Total Fat: 2.1 g, Total Carbs: 1.3 g, Protein: 5.3 g.

18. Miso and Tofu With Sesame Glaze and Sautéed Vegetables in a Pan With Ginger and Chili

Preparation time: 20 minutes - Cooking time: 10 minutes - Servings: 1

- 2 teaspoons of extra virgin olive oil
- 7 ounces of mushrooms (enoki or champignon)
- ½ carrot, peeled and cut into julienne strips
- 1 red chili peppers, sliced
- 1 tablespoon of fresh ginger
- Cabbage or spinach
- Onion
- Miso paste
- 125 g of tofu

1. In a large pan, heat the oil and add the mushrooms and carrot to it. Quickly cook the vegetables for 1minute or as long as they are tender, add the chili, the ginger and cook for 10 seconds.

2. Add the cabbage or spinach and ì onions in the pan and cook until the leaves are slightly wilted. Remove them from the pans and divide them into two bowls.

3. Bring 700 ml of water to the boiling point in a large saucepan. Mix the miso with a few teaspoons of water in a small bowl and add it to the pot. Stir to mix and still incorporate miso if necessary. Divide the drained and diced tofu into the bowls and cover with the miso broth. Add tamari or soy sauce and serve immediately.

Nutrition: Calories: 114, Sodium: 7.3 mg, Dietary Fiber: 2.4 g, Total Fat: 2.1 g, Total Carbs: 1.3 g, Protein: 5.3 g.

19. Blueberry Banana Pancakes

Preparation time: 10 minutes - Cooking time: 10 minutes - Servings: 1

- 3 bananas
- 3 eggs
- 75 g rolled oats
- A pinch of salt
- 1 teaspoon baking powder
- ¾ cup of blueberries (fresh or frozen)

1. To complete this recipe, you will need to do the following:

2. Put your oats into a blender or food processor and pulse until you have created an oat flour.

3. In your food processor or blender, add in everything but the blueberries. Pulse it together for roughly 2 minutes until it is well combined and you have a nice, smooth batter.

4. Pour the batter into a large mixing bowl and gently add in the blueberries, folding them in rather than mixing it up. Make sure that you do not overmix.

5. Wait 10 minutes, allowing the baking powder to activate.

6. Heat a medium-high frying pan and add a tiny amount of oil or butter to the surface so that the pancake does not stick. Scoop in the blueberry banana batter to the size desired and allowed it to fry until the bottom is golden brown and ready to flip.

7. Flip and cook the other side until also golden brown.

Nutrition: Calories: 495 Sodium: 32 mg Dietary Fiber: 1.4 g Total Fat: 2.6 g Total Carbs: 12.3 g Protein: 1.3 g

20. Breakfast Chocolate Muffins

Preparation time: 10 minutes - Cooking time: 30 minutes - Servings: 1

- Almond paste
- Banana (Blackberry)
- 1 Egg
- 1 Teaspoon vanilla extract
- 1/2 teaspoon tartar yeast
- 100 grams of chocolate chips

1. To prepare a baking tray made of paper or silicone muffins, preheat the oven to 200 ° C.

2. Put all ingredients (except optional chocolate chips) in a food processor and mix it in a smooth, sticky dough.

3. Optional: add and mix chocolate bars

4. Optional: add and incorporate chocolate bars

5. Place the dough in a muffin pan and bake until golden, then cook for about 12-15 minutes.

Nutrition: Calories: 205 Sodium: 32 mg Dietary Fiber: 1.5 g Total Fat: 5.1 g Total Carbs: 16.4 g Protein: 1.3 g

21. Cauliflower Couscous

Preparation time: 20 minutes - Cooking time: 10 minutes - Servings: 1

- 28-ounces cauliflower
- 7 dried tomatoes
- 1 tablespoon of capers
- 1 anchovy in oil
- 2 tablespoons of pitted Taggiasca olives
- 1 clove of garlic
- 7 ounces of marinated anchovies
- Fresh oregano
- Extra virgin olive oil

1. To prepare the cauliflower couscous, remove the leaves and remove the florets. Rinse the couscous under running freshwater, dab them with kitchen paper to dry them and blend them, a little at a time, in a food processor and transfer the granules obtained in a clean bowl.

2. Let the dried tomatoes soak in lukewarm water for half an hour, then squeeze them, dab them with paper towels and cut them into thin strips. Drain the capers and chop half of them with a knife. Coarsely chop also half of the olives. Peel the garlic and use the palm of your hand to mash it. In a large pan, heat a little oil. Fry the garlic with the capers (chopped and whole), the anchovy, and the chopped olives. Also, add the sliced tomatoes over high heat.

3. Pour the cauliflower grains and stir in with a little water (about half a glass: the cauliflower must remain crunchy), always on high heat, and stir. Add salt, turn off the heat and

add the anchovies marinated in fillets, the remaining olives, a little fresh oregano leaves and a round of raw oil.

4. Serve the cauliflower couscous, hot or cold, depending on your taste.

Nutrition: Calories: 114, Sodium: 7.3 mg, Dietary Fiber: 2.4 g, Total Fat: 2.1 g, Total Carbs: 1.3 g, Protein: 5.3 g.

22. *Turkey Escalopes With Sage, Parsley, and Capers*

Preparation time: 20 minutes - Cooking time: 10 minutes - Servings: 1

- 8 slices of turkey
- Half white onion
- 1 large sprig of parsley
- A few fresh sage leaves or a nice pinch of the dried one
- Olive oil to taste
- Salt
- Capers
- Flour

1. Cover the turkey slices with flour once at the time, shake them slightly to remove excess flour. Wash parsley, sage, and finely chop them with a knife, add the capers. Finely chop the onion, heat up 2 tablespoons of oil in a pan, add the onion, fry 1 minute, add 2 tablespoons of water, lower the heat, cover and cook the onion, add 3 tablespoons of oil, raise the heat, put on the heat the slices of turkey in the pan, brown them on both sides, salt.

2. One minute before turning off the heat, sprinkle the slices with the chopped sage and parsley with capers. Serve with the sauce made from the pan.

Nutrition: Calories: 120, Sodium: 23 mg, Dietary Fiber: 2.4 g, Total Fat: 2.1 g, Total Carbs: 1.3 g, Protein: 10.3 g.

23. *Cabbage and Red Onion Dahl With Buckwheat*

Preparation time: 20 minutes - Cooking time: 30 minutes - Servings: 1

- 7.5-ounces hulled buckwheat
- 1.5ounces of curly cabbage
- Vegetable broth
- 1 Tomato pulp
- 2 spoons of extra virgin olive oil
- Red onion
- Basil
- Chopped chili pepper
- Water
- Pepper
- Salt

1. Into a kettle, pour the water, add the oil and, to the fire, wait until it boils and add the broth. Then turn off the heat. Meanwhile, wash the cauliflower, cut the florets into small pieces and drain them. Chop the shallot finely enough. Pour the buckwheat in a colander and rinse it under running water.

2. In another saucepan (large) pour two full spoons of oil, add the chopped shallot, the mince for sautéing and fry it on a soft flame, often mixing to prevent it from sticking to the pot. When the onion is transparent and dried, add the buckwheat and toast it for a few minutes, mixing without letting it stick to the bottom of the pot. Then add the tomato pulp, broth, chopped basil, chopped red pepper, and mix, then add the cauliflower florets.

3. Cook the Buckwheat and cauliflower soup for 30 minutes, covering the pan with a lid and on low heat, occasionally stirring so as not to stick the buckwheat to the pan. If necessary, season with salt. After cooking, serve the buckwheat and cauliflower soup with freshly ground pepper. If you like (and if you are not vegan, vegetarian or lactose intolerant), you could also add some grated pecorino cheese. Your buckwheat and cauliflower soup is ready!

Nutrition: Calories: 120, Sodium: 23 mg, Dietary Fiber: 2.4 g, Total Fat: 2.1 g, Total Carbs: 1.3 g, Protein: 10.3 g.

24. *Mushroom and Tofu Scramble*

Preparation time: 10 minutes - Cooking time: 20 minutes - Servings: 2

- 7 ounces of extra firm tofu
- 2 teaspoon turmeric powder
- 1 teaspoon black pepper
- 1.50ounces of kale, roughly chopped
- 2 teaspoon extra virgin olive oil
- 1.5 ounces of red onion, thinly sliced
- 1 Thai chilies, thinly sliced
- 100g mushrooms, thinly sliced
- 4 tablespoons parsley, finely chopped

1. To help it drain, cover the tofu in paper towels and put something heavy on top.

2. Mix the turmeric with a little water until you achieve a light paste.

3. Steam the kale for 2 to 3 minutes.

4. Heat the olive oil over medium heat in a frying pan until hot but not smoky, add the onion, chili, and mushrooms and fry for 2 to 3 minutes until they have started to brown and soften.

5. Crumble the tofu and return to the pan into bite-size bits, pour the turmeric paste over the tofu, and mix thoroughly. Add the black pepper and stir. Cook over medium heat for 2 to 3 minutes, so the spices are cooked through and the tofu has started to brown.

6. Attach the kale and continue cooking for another minute, over medium heat. Finally, blend well, add the parsley, and serve.

Nutrition: Calories: 123 Sodium: 36 mg Dietary Fiber: 2.4 g Total Fat: 4.7 g Total Carbs: 16.3 g Protein: 1.3 g

25. *Kale Scramble*

Preparation time: 10 minutes - Cooking time: 6 minutes - Total time: 16 minutes - Servings: 2

- 4 eggs
- 1/8 teaspoon ground turmeric
- Salt and ground black pepper, to taste
- 1 tablespoon water
- 2 teaspoons olive oil
- 1 cup fresh kale, tough ribs removed and chopped

1. In a bowl, add the eggs, turmeric, salt, black pepper, and water and with a whisk, beat until foamy.

2. In a wok, over medium heat, heat the oil.

3. Add the egg mixture and stir to combine.

4. Reduce the heat to medium-low right away and cook for about 1– 2 minutes, stirring frequently.

5. Stir in the kale and cook for 3 to 4 minutes or so, stirring frequently.

6. Remove from the heat and serve immediately.

Nutrition: Calories: 183 Sodium: 35 mg Dietary Fiber: 2.4 g Total Fat: 4.1 g Total Carbs: 16.8 g Protein: 1.6 g

26. Green Omelet

Preparation Time: 5 Minutes - **Cooking Time:** 35 Minutes - **Servings:** 1

- 1 tsp of olive oil
- 1 shallot peeled and finely chopped 2 large eggs
- Salt and freshly ground black pepper A handful of parsley, finely chopped A handful of rocket

Heat the oil in a large frying pan, over medium-low heat. Add the shallot and gently fry for about 5 minutes. Increase the heat and cook for two more minutes.

In a cup or bowl, whisk the eggs; distribute the shallot in the pan then add in the eggs. Evenly distribute the eggs by tipping over the pan on all sides. Cook for about a minute before lifting the sides and allowing the runny eggs to move to the base of the pan.

Sprinkle rocket leaves and parsley on top and season with pepper and salt to taste.

When the base is just starting to brown, tip it onto a plate and serve right away.

Nutrition Facts: Calories 221 kcal, Fat 28 g, Carbohydrate 10.6 g, Protein 9.5 g

27. Apple Blackcurrant Compote Pancakes

Preparation time: 5 minutes - **Cooking time:** 15 minutes - **Servings:** 4

For the compote:

- 3s of water 2s caster sugar
- 120 grams blackcurrants, washed and stalks removed

For The Apple Pancakes:

- 2 teaspoons light olive oil 2 egg whites 300 ml semi-skimmed milk 2 apples, cut into small pieces
- Pinch of salt
- 2s of caster sugar
- 1 teaspoon of baking powder 125 grams plain flour
- 75 grams porridge oats

In a small pan, add the blackcurrants, water and sugar. Bring it to a boil and let it simmer for 10 to 15 minutes.

In a large bowl, place the flour, oats, baking powder, salt and caster sugar, mix well.

Add in the apple, stir and gently fold in semi-skimmed milk until mixture is smooth.

Beat the egg whites until firm peaks are formed, then gently whisk them into the mixture of flour. Pour batter into a jug.

Heat half teaspoon of oil over medium-high heat in a non-stick frying pan. Add about 1/4 of the batter into the pan. Cook pancake until golden brown on both sides. Drizzle the blackcurrant compote.

Nutrition: Calories: 337 Net carbs: 40 g Fat: 9.82g Fiber: 6.2 g Protein: 32g

28. Blueberry Oats Pancakes

Preparation time: 5 minutes - **Cooking time:** 5 minutes - **Servings:** 4

- 225 grams blueberries
- ¼ teaspoon salt
- 2 teaspoon baking powder
- 150 grams rolled oats
- 6 eggs
- 6 bananas

Pulse the rolled oats for 1 minute in a (dry) high-speed blender to form oat flour.

Add in the eggs, bananas, salt and baking powder and process for 2 minutes until it forms a smooth batter.

Pour the batter into a big bowl and add the blueberries, stirring gently. Let sit for at least 10 minutes to activate the baking powder.

Over a medium high heat, add a big spoonful of butter to the frying pan.

Scoop the batter and cook until nicely golden underneath. Flip pancake and cook the other side.

Nutrition: Calories: 494 Net carbs: 68 g Fat: 11.3g Fiber: 6.2 g Protein: 22.23g

29. Muesli Yoghurt Breakfast

Preparation time: 3 minutes - **Cooking time:** 0 minutes - **Servings:** 1

- 100g plain Greek, coconut or soya yoghurt 100g hulled and chopped strawberries
- 10g cocoa nibs
- 15g chopped walnuts
- 40g pitted and chopped Medjool dates 15g coconut flakes
- 10g buckwheat puffs 20g buckwheat flakes

Mix together the cocoa nibs, buckwheat flakes, coconut flakes, buckwheat puffs, Medjool dates and walnuts. Add the yoghurt and strawberries.

Nutrition: Calories: 368 Net carbs: 49g Fat: 11.5g Fiber: 7.4g Protein: 16.54g

30. Omelette Fold

Preparation time: 3 minutes - **Cooking time:** 5 minutes - **Servings:** 1

- 1 teaspoon extra virgin olive oil
- 5 grams thinly sliced parsley 35 grams thinly sliced red chicory 3 medium eggs
- 50 grams streaky bacon, cut into thin strips

Cook the bacon strips in hot non-stick frying pan over high heat until crispy.

Remove and drain any excess fat on a kitchen paper.

Beat the eggs in a small bowl and mix with the parsley and chicory. Mix the drained bacon through the egg mixture.

In a non-stick pan, heat the olive oil; add the mixture. Cook until omelette is set. Loose the omelette around the edges with a spatula and fold into half- moon.

Nutrition: Calories: 471 Net carbs: 3.3g Fat: 38.72g Fiber: 1.5g Protein: 27g

31. Cherry Tomatoes Red Pesto Porridge

Preparation Time: 10 minutes - **Cooking Time:** 5 minutes - **Servings:** 2

- Salt, pepper 1 teaspoon hemp seed 1 teaspoon pumpkin seed 2 teaspoons nutritional yeast ½ cup couscous ½ cup oats
- 1 teaspoon sun-dried tomato-walnut pesto 1 teaspoon tahini
- 1 tablespoon callion 1 cup sliced cherry tomatoes 1 cup chopped kale 1 teaspoon dried basil 1.5 teaspoon dried oregano 2 cups veggie stock

In a small cooking pot, add oats, oregano, vegetable stock, basil, couscous, Pepper and salt and cook on medium heat for around 5 minutes, stirring regularly, until the porridge is creamy and fluffy.

Add chopped kale but reserve a bit for garnish, tomatoes and sliced scallion. Cook for additional 1 minute, stir in pesto, tahini, and nutritional yeast. Top with the reserved kale, pumpkin and hemp seeds plus cherry tomatoes.
Nutrition: Calories: 259 Net carbs: 36g Fat: 7.68g Fiber: 7.4g Protein: 14.26g

32. Sautéed Veggies Bowl
Preparation time: 5 minutes - Cooking time: 5 minutes - Servings: 1
For tofu scramble:
- 1 cup water
- Dash of soy sauce Pepper and salt
- 1 teaspoon turmeric
- 1 serving medium crumbled firm tofu For the Sautéed Veggies:
- 1/2 cup red onions, diced 1 cup mushrooms, sliced
- 1 big handful kale, de-stemmed and chopped

For the Bowls
- 1/2 cup cooked brown rice 1/2 avocado, pitted

Mix together the tofu scramble ingredients in a small dish, set aside. Add a splash of water in a skillet over medium-high heat; add the onions, mushrooms and kale. Cook, stirring periodically, for about 5-8 minutes or until it is evenly brown and soft. Set aside in a bowl.
Using the same skillet, pour in the tofu mixture and cook until it starts to brown and heated through for 5 minutes. Transfer tofu scramble into a bowl, add the mushrooms/kale mixture, top with avocado, brown rice and salsa. Serve with flatbreads, buckwheat, basmati rice or couscous.
Nutrition: Calories: 122g Fats: 6.9g Sodium 867g Net carbs: 8.7g Fiber: 1.7g Sugar: 4.9g Protein: 7.3g

33. Chocolate Oats Granola
Preparation time: 10 minutes - Cooking time: 20 minutes - Servings: 8
- 60 grams good-quality dark chocolate chips (70%) 2 of rice malt syrup or maple syrup
- 1 tablespoon dark brown sugar 20g roughly chopped butter
- 3 teaspoons light olive oil 50g roughly chopped pecans
- 200g of jumbo oats
- Heat-up your oven to 160°C).

In a large bowl, mix together pecan and oats. Gently heat the butter, olive oil, rice malt syrup and brown sugar in a small non-stick pan until the sugar and syrup is dissolved and butter melted. Do not allow the mixture boil before removing. Spread the mixture on top the oats and stir very well to coat with the oats.
Distribute the oats mixture onto a large parchment lined baking tray, spread out into every corners. You do not need to spread evenly, leave lumps of mixture with spacing.
Place tray in the oven and bake until edges are just tinged golden brown, about 20 minutes. Withdraw from the oven and let completely cool on the tray.
Once cool, use your finger to break up any lager lumps. Add in the chocolate chips and mix. Serve Chocolate granola with cup of green tea.
Nutrition: Calories: 244 Net carbs: 20.91g Fat: 15.41g Fiber: 4.6 g Protein: 5.24g

34. Green Chia Spinach Pudding
Preparation Time: 30 minutes - Cooking Time: 0 minutes - Servings: 1
- 3 spoons of chia seeds 1 Medjool date, slice in half and remove pit 1 handful fresh spinach 1 cup non-dairy milk Toppings Banana, berries, etc.

Blend the spinach, date and milk in a high speed blender until very smooth. Pour the mixture in a bowl over the chia seeds. Stir mixture well, and stirring every now and then for about 15 minutes.
Transfer to the refrigerator and give at least one hour or overnight to chill.Stir once more, just before serving; top with kiwi, banana, berries, etc.
Nutrition: Calories: 232g Fats: 9.6g Sodium 86mg Net Carbs: 2.6g Fiber: 9.9g Protein 10.1g

35. Blackcurrant and Raspberry Breakfast
Preparation time: 5 minutes - Cooking time: 15 minutes - Servings: 2
- 300 ml water 2 teaspoons granulated sugar
- 100 grams blackcurrants, washed and stalks removed 2 leaves gelatin 100 grams raspberries, washed

In two serving glasses, add the raspberries and set aside.
Add cold water in a bowl and place the gelatin leaves to soften.
In a small pan, add the blackcurrants with 100 ml of water along with the sugar. Bring to the boil. Enable it to boil for five minutes, then turn off the heat. Remove and cool for 2 minutes.
Remove the gelatin leaves and squeeze out excess water. Place leaves in the saucepan. Stir continuously until fully dissolved, add and stir together in the remaining water. Pour liquid over raspberries in the glasses or dishes. Place for around 3-4 hours or overnight in the refrigerator and allow to set.
Nutrition: Calories: 76 Net carbs: 13.57g Fat: 0.5g Fiber: 3.3 g Protein: 4g

36. Kale Mushroom Scramble
Preparation time: 10 minutes - Cooking time: 6 minutes - Servings: 1
- 5g of finely chopped parsley
- Handful of thinly sliced button mushrooms
- ½ thinly sliced bird's eye chili 1 teaspoon extra virgin olive oil 20g kale, roughly chopped
- 1 teaspoon mild curry powder
- 1 teaspoon ground turmeric 2 eggs

Mix together the curry powder, turmeric and a small splash of water to form a light paste. Add the kale to a steamer basket and steam in boiling water for 2– 3 minutes. Heat the oil over medium heat in a frying pan and fry mushrooms and chili for 2 to 3 minutes until soften and starting to brown.
Nutrition: Calories: 116g Fats: 5.4g Net carbs: 13.2g Fiber: 3.6g Proteins 5.8g

37. Walnut Medjool Porridge
Preparation time: 10 minutes - Cooking time: 15 minutes - Servings: 1
- 50g strawberries, hulled 1 teaspoon walnut butter 35g Buckwheat flakes
- 1 chopped Medjool date

- 200 ml almond or coconut milk, unsweetened

Add the date and milk into a frying pan over medium low heat, then add in the flakes and cook to your desired consistency.

Add in the walnut butter, stir well. Top porridge with strawberries.

Nutrition: Calories: 550 Net carbs: 25g Fat: 45g Fiber: 9 g Protein: 6.57g

38. *Avocado Tofu Breakfast Salad*

Preparation Time: 5 minutes - Cooking time: 5 minutes - Servings: 1

- Half a lemon juice Half a red onion, chopped 2 tomatoes, chopped One spoon chili sauce 4 handfuls baby spinach
- A handful of chopped almonds 1 pink chopped grapefruit
- 1 Avocado, chopped Half a pack of firm tofu, chopped 2 Tortillas

Heat the tortillas in the oven for 8 to 10 minutes.

Combine tomatoes, tofu and onions with some chili sauce in a bowl, place inside the refrigerator to cool.

Add the avocado, grapefruit and almonds. Mix everything together and place into the bowl.

Top with a Squeeze of fresh lemon juice!

Nutrition: Calories 94g Fats 2.1g Net Carbs 11.3gProtein 3.9g

39. *Buckwheat Coconut Overnight Porridge*

Preparation time: 10 minutes - Cooking time: 8 minutes - Servings: 4-6

- 1/4 teaspoon of cinnamon 2 teaspoon of vanilla extract 1 cup water 3 cups unsweetened coconut, soy or almond milk 1/4 cup chia seeds 1 cup of buckwheat groats (not kasha) Pinch of salt For the Toppings:
- 1 1/2 cup berries 1/2 cup walnuts

In a bowl, combine together the buckwheat groats, coconut milk, chia seeds, cinnamon, water, vanilla extract and salt. Cover bowl with stretch film, transfer to the fridge and let sit overnight.

Bring it out in the morning and place it in a pot; cook mixture in the pot for 10-12 minutes, stirring occasionally until your desired thickness is reached. Add the toppings and Serve.

Nutrition: Calories: 400 Net carbs: 47g Fat: 17.55g Fiber: 3.7g Protein: 11.19g

40. *Strawberry and Cherry Smoothie*

Preparation time: 10 minutes - Cooking time: 0 minutes - Servings: 1

- 100g strawberries
- 75g frozen pitted cherries 1 cup plain full-fat yogurt 175mls unsweetened soya milk

In a blender, put all of the ingredients and process until smooth.

Nutrition: Calories: 132 Fats: 1.5g Net Carbs: 28.4g Fiber: 2.9g Proteins 2.9g

41. *Banana Snap*

Preparation time: 10 minutes - Cooking time: 0 minutes - Servings: 1

- 2.5cm chunk fresh ginger, peeled 1 banana 1 large carrot
- 1 apple, cored ½ stick of celery ¼ level teaspoon turmeric powder

With just enough water to cover them, put all the ingredients in a blender. Process until smooth

Nutrition: Calories: 34 Net carbs: 7.8g Fat: 0.1g Fiber: 3.7g Protein: 2g

42. *Green Egg Scramble*

Preparation time: 5 minutes - Cooking time: 5 minutes - Servings: 1

- 2 eggs, whisked
- 25g rocket (arugula) leaves 10g chives, chopped
- 10g teaspoon fresh basil, chopped 10g teaspoon fresh parsley, chopped 1 teaspoon olive oil

Mix the eggs together with the rocket (arugula) and herbs. Heat the oil in a frying pan and pour into the egg mixture. Gently stir until it's lightly scrambled. Season and serve.

Nutrition: Calories: 101 Net carbs: 2.1g Fat: 7g Fiber: 0.5g Protein: 7.1g

43. *Green Sirtfood Smoothie*

Preparation time: 10 minutes - Cooking time: 0 minutes - Servings: 1

- 100g unsweetened
- Greek yoghurt
- 6 walnut halves
- 8-10 medium strawberries
- A handful of kale leaves
- 20g dark chocolate (min. 85% cocoa)
- 1 date
- 1/2 teaspoon turmeric S
- mall piece fresh chili, finely chopped
- 200ml unsweetened almond milk

Put it all in a blender and combine until you get a smoothie.

Nutrition: Calories: 72 Net carbs: 14g Fat: 0.3g Fiber: 0.8g Protein: 2.8g

44. *Power Cereals*

Preparation time: 10 minutes - Cooking time: 0 minutes - Servings: 1

- 20g buckwheat flakes 10g puffed buckwheat 15g coconut flakes
- 40g Medjool dates, seeded and chopped 10g cocoa nibs
- 100g strawberries
- 100g Greek natural yoghurt

Mix all ingredients together.

Nutrition: Calories: 124g Net carbs: 27.4g Fat: 1.1g Fiber: 1.7g Protein: 2.3g

45. *Berry Yoghurt*

Preparation time: 10 minutes - Cooking time: 0 minutes - Servings: 1

- 125g mixed berries 150g Greek yoghurt 25g walnuts, chopped 10g dark chocolate (85%)

Simply mix all ingredients together.

Nutrition: Calories: 115 Net carbs: 22.5g Fat: 1.2g Fiber: 1.1g Protein: 3g

46. Blueberry Frozen Yogurt

Preparation time: 1 hour 10 minutes - Cooking time: 0 minutes - Servings: 4

- 1 teaspoon honey
- 450g plain yogurt 175g blueberries Juice of 1 orange

Place the blueberries and orange juice into a food processor or blender and blitz until smooth. In a large cup, press the mixture through a sieve to extract the seeds. Stir in the honey and yogurt. Transfer the mixture to an ice-cream maker and follow the manufacturer's instructions. Alternatively pour the mixture into a container and place in the fridge for 1 hour. Use a fork to whisk it and break up ice crystals and freeze for 2 hours.

Nutrition: Calories: 66 Net carbs: 8.3g Protein: 8.2g

47. Vegetable & Nut Loaf

Preparation time: 15 minutes - Cooking time: 1 hour 45 minutes - Servings: 4

- 175g mushrooms, finely chopped
- 100g haricot beans
- 100g walnuts, finely chopped 100g peanuts, finely chopped 1 carrot, finely chopped
- 3 sticks celery, finely chopped
- 1 bird's-eye chili, finely chopped 1 red onion, finely chopped
- 1 egg, beaten
- 2 cloves garlic, chopped 2 teaspoons olive oil
- 2 teaspoons turmeric powder 2teaspoonss soy sauce 4g fresh parsley, chopped 100mls water
- 60mls red wine

In a pan, heat the oil and add the garlic, chili, carrot, celery, onion, mushrooms and turmeric. Cook for 5 minutes. Place the haricot beans in a bowl and stir in the nuts, vegetables, soy sauce, egg, parsley, red wine and water. Grease a wide loaf tin with greaseproof paper and line it.Spoon the mixture into the loaf tin, cover with foil and bake in the oven at 190C/375F for 60-90 minutes. Let it stand on a serving plate for 10 minutes, then turn it on.

Nutrition: Calories: 280 Net carbs: 29.7g Fat: 16.3g Fiber: 1.2g Protein: 4.6g

48. Dates & Parma Ham

Preparation time: 15 minutes - Cooking time: 0 minutes - Servings: 4

- 12 medjool dates
- 2 slices Parma ham, cut into strips

Wrap each date with a Parma ham strip. Can be served hot or cold.

Nutrition: Calories: 202 Net carbs: 17.9g Protein: 0.4G

49. Braised Celery

Preparation time: 15 minutes - Cooking time: 15 minutes - Servings: 4

- 250g celery, chopped
- 100mls warm vegetable stock (broth) 1 red onion, chopped 1 clove of garlic, crushed 1 fresh parsley, chopped 25g butter Sea salt and freshly ground black pepper

Place the celery, onion, stock (broth) and garlic into a saucepan and bring it to the boil, lower the heat and let it simmer for 10 minutes. Stir in the parsley and butter and season with salt and pepper. Serve as an accompaniment to roast meat dishes.

Nutrition: Calories: 367 Net carbs: 5.9g Fat: 0.2g Fiber: 2.4g Protein: 1.2g

50. Cheesy Buckwheat Cakes

Preparation time: 15 minutes - Cooking time: 10 minutes - Servings: 2

- 100g buckwheat, cooked and cooled
- 1 large egg 25g cheddar cheese, grated (shredded)
- 25g (1oz) whole meal breadcrumbs
- 2 shallots, chopped 2 s fresh parsley, chopped 1 olive oil

Crack the bowl with the egg, whisk it, and set it aside. In a separate bowl combine all the buckwheat, cheese, shallots and parsley and mix well.

Pour in the beaten egg to the buckwheat mixture and stir well. Shape the mixture into patties. Scatter the breadcrumbs on a plate and roll the patties in them. Heat the olive oil in a large frying pan and gently place the cakes in the oil. Cook until slightly golden on either side for 3-4 minutes.

Nutrition: Calories: 358 Net carbs: 121.5g Fat: 5,7g Fiber: 17g Protein: 22.5g

51. Soy Berry Smoothie

Preparation time: 5 minutes. - **Cooking time:** 0 minutes. - **Serving:** 1

- 1 cup fresh strawberries/blueberries or frozen
- 1 cup unsweetened vanilla soymilk

Blend or blitz all the ingredients. Enjoy.

Nutrition: Calories: 260cal Carbs: 44g Sugar: 34g Fat: 4.5g

52. Paleolicious Smoothie Bowl

Preparation time: 5 minutes. - **Cooking time:** 0 minutes. - **Serving:** 1

- 1 piece banana (frozen)
- 1 hand spinach
- 1/2 pieces mango
- 1/2 pieces avocado
- 100 milliliters almond milk
- ½ pieces mango
- 1 hand raspberries
- 1 tablespoon grated coconut
- 1 tablespoon walnuts, roughly chopped

1. In a blender, place the ingredients and combine to an even mass
2. Put the mixture in a bowl and garnish with the remaining ingredients.
3. Of course, you can vary the garnish as you wish.

Nutrition: Calories: 180cal Carbs: 42g Sugar: 30g Fat: 31.5g

53. Banana-Peanut Butter 'n Greens Smoothie

Preparation time: 5 minutes. - **Cooking time:** 0 minutes. - **Servings:** 1

- 1 cup chopped and packed Romaine lettuce
- 1 frozen medium banana
- 1 tablespoon all-natural peanut butter
- 1 cup cold almond milk

1. In a heavy-duty blender, add all the ingredients.
2. Puree until smooth and creamy.
3. Serve and enjoy.

Nutrition: Calories: 349.3cal   Fat: 9.7g   Carbs: 57.4g
Protein: 8.1g

54. Fruity Tofu Smoothie
Preparation time: 5 minutes. - **Cooking time:** 0 minutes. - **Servings:** 2
- 1 cup ice-cold water
- 1 cup packed spinach
- ¼ cup frozen mango chunks
- ½ cup frozen pineapple chunks
- 1 tablespoon chia seeds
- 1 container silken tofu
- 1 frozen medium banana

1. Add all of the ingredients into a blender until smooth and fluffy.
2. Evenly divide into two glasses, serve, and enjoy.
Nutrition: Calories: 175cal   Fat: 3.7g   Carbs: 33.3g
Protein: 6.0g

55. Green Vegetable Smoothie
Preparation time: 5 minutes. - **Cooking time:** 0 minutes. - **Servings:** 4
- 1 cup cold water
- ½ cup strawberries
- 2 ounces baby spinach
- 1 lemon juice
- 1 tablespoon fresh mint
- 1 banana
- ½ cup blueberries

1. Put the ingredients in a blender.
Nutrition: Calories: 52cal Fat: 2g Carbs: 12g
Protein: 1g

56. Creamy Oats, Greens & Blueberry Smoothie
Preparation time: 4 minutes. - **Cooking time:** 0 minutes. - **Servings:** 1
- 1 cup cold fat-free milk
- 1 cup salad greens
- ½ cup fresh frozen blueberries
- ½ cup frozen cooked oatmeal
- 1 tablespoon sunflower seeds

1. In a blender, put all the ingredients until smooth and creamy.
Nutrition: Calories: 280cal   Fat: 6.8g   Carbs: 44.0g
Protein: 14.0g

57. Potato Bites
Preparation time: 10 minutes. - **Cooking time:** 20 minutes. - **Servings:** 4
- 1 potato, sliced
- 2 bacon slices, already cooked and crumbled
- 1 small avocado, pitted and cubed
- Cooking spray

1. Spread potato slices on a lined baking sheet, spray with cooking oil, introduce in the oven at 350°F, bake for 20 minutes, arrange on a platter, top each slice with avocado and crumbled bacon and serve as a snack.
Nutrition: Calories: 180cal Fat: 4g Fiber: 1g Carbs: 8g
Protein: 6g

58. Sesame Dip
Preparation time: 10 minutes. - **Cooking time:** 0 minutes. - **Servings:** 4
- 1 cup sesame seed paste, pure
- Black pepper to taste
- 1 cup veggie stock
- ½ cup lemon juice
- ½ teaspoon cumin, ground
- 3 garlic cloves, chopped

1. In your food processor, mix the sesame paste with black pepper, stock, lemon juice, cumin and garlic, pulse very well, divide into bowls and serve as a party dip.
Nutrition: Calories: 120cal Fat: 12g Fiber: 2g Carbs: 7g
Protein: 4g

59. Rosemary Squash Dip
Preparation time: 10 minutes. - **Cooking time:** 40 minutes. - **Servings:** 4
- 1 cup butternut squash, peeled and cubed
- 1 tablespoon water
- Cooking spray
- 2 tablespoons coconut milk
- 2 teaspoons rosemary, dried
- Black pepper to taste

1. Spread squash cubes on a lined baking sheet, spray some cooking oil, introduce in the oven, bake at 365°F for 40 minutes, transfer to your blender, add water, milk, rosemary and black pepper, pulse well, divide into small bowls and serve.
Nutrition: Calories: 182cal Fat: 5g Fiber: 7g Carbs: 12g
Protein: 5g

60. Bean Spread
Preparation time: 10 minutes. - **Cooking time:** 7 hours. - **Servings:** 4
- 1 cup white beans, dried
- 1 teaspoon apple cider vinegar
- 1 cup veggie stock
- 1 tablespoon water

1. In your slow cooker, mix beans with stock, stir, cover, cook over low heat for 6 hours, drain, transfer to your food processor, add vinegar and water, pulse well, divide into bowls and serve.
Nutrition: Calories: 181cal Fat: 6g Fiber: 5g Carbs: 9g
Protein: 7g

61. Carrots and Cauliflower Spread
Preparation time: 10 minutes. - **Cooking time:** 40 minutes. - **Servings:** 4
- 1 cup carrots, sliced
- 2 cups cauliflower florets
- ½ cup cashews
- 2 (½) cups water
- 1 cup almond milk
- 1 teaspoon garlic powder
- ¼ teaspoon smoked paprika

1. In a small pot, mix the carrots with cauliflower, cashews and water, stir, cover, bring to a boil over medium heat, cook for 40 minutes, drain and transfer to a blender.
2. Add almond milk, garlic powder and paprika, pulse well, divide into small bowls and serve.
Nutrition: Calories: 201cal Fat: 7g Fiber: 4g Carbs: 7g
Protein: 7g

62. Italian Veggie Salsa

Preparation time: 10 minutes. - **Cooking time:** 10 minutes. - **Servings:** 4

- 2 red bell peppers, cut into medium wedges
- 3 zucchinis, sliced
- ½ cup garlic, minced
- 2 tablespoons olive oil
- A pinch of black pepper
- 1 teaspoon Italian seasoning

1. Heat a pan with the oil over medium-high heat, add bell peppers and zucchini, toss and cook for 5 minutes.
2. Add garlic, black pepper and Italian seasoning, toss, cook for 5 minutes more, divide into small cups and serve as a snack.

Nutrition: Calories: 132cal Fat: 3g Fiber: 3g Carbs: 7g Protein:4g

63. Sweet Oatmeal

Preparation Time: 5 minutes - **Cooking Time**: 10 minutes - **Servings:** 3

- 1 cup oatmeal
- 5 apricots
- 1 tablespoon honey
- 1 cup coconut milk, unsweetened
- 1 teaspoon cashew butter
- ¼ teaspoon salt
- ½ cup of water

1. Combine the coconut milk and oatmeal together in the saucepan and stir the mixture.
2. Add the water and stir it again. Sprinkle the mixture with the salt and close the lid.
3. Cook the oatmeal on medium heat for 10 minutes.
4. Meanwhile, chop the apricots into tiny pieces and combine the chopped fruit with the honey.
5. When the oatmeal is cooked, add cashew butter and fruit mixture.
6. Stir carefully and transfer to serving bowls.
7. Serve immediately.

Nutrition: Calories: 336, Fat: 21.2g, Total Carbs: 35.1g, Sugars: 14.0g, Protein: 6.2g

64. Green Beans and Eggs

Preparation Time: 10 minutes - **Cooking Time**: 15 minutes - **Servings:** 2

- ½ cup green beans
- ¼ teaspoon salt
- 5 eggs
- 1/3 cup skim milk
- 1 bell pepper, seeds removed
- 1 teaspoon olive oil

1. Slice the bell pepper and combine it with the green beans.
2. Pour the olive oil in a skillet and transfer the vegetable mixture to the skillet.
3. Cook for 3 minutes over medium heat, stirring frequently. Meanwhile, beat the eggs in a mixing bowl.
4. Sprinkle the egg mixture with the salt and add skim milk. Whisk well.
5. Pour the egg mixture over the vegetable mixture and cook for 3 minutes on medium heat.
6. Stir the mixture carefully so that the eggs and vegetables are well combined.
7. Cook for 4 minutes more.

8. Stir again and close the lid.
9. Cook the scrambled eggs for 5 minutes more.
10. Stir the mixture again.

Nutrition: Calories: 231, Fat: 13.4g, Total Carbs: 9.3g, Sugars: 6.2g, Protein:16.3g

65. Spiced Morning Omelet

Preparation Time: 10 minutes - **Cooking Time**: 15 minutes - **Servings**: 3

- 7 eggs
- 1/3 cup skim milk
- 3 garlic cloves
- ¼ teaspoon nutmeg
- ¼ teaspoon ground ginger
- 1 teaspoon cilantro
- 1 teaspoon olive oil
- 1 tablespoon chives
- 1 teaspoon turmeric

1. Beat the eggs in a mixing bowl.
2. Add the skim milk and whisk again.
3. Sprinkle the egg mixture with the nutmeg, ground ginger, cilantro, and turmeric.
4. Peel the garlic cloves and mince them.
5. Chop the chives and combine with the minced garlic.
6. Add the herb mixture to the eggs and stir it again.
7. Preheat a skillet well and pour in the olive oil.
8. Preheat the olive oil over medium heat and then pour the egg mixture into the pan.
9. Close the lid and cook the omelet for 15 minutes.
10. When the dish is cooked, cool slightly and cut into the serving portions.

Nutrition: Calories: 179, Fat: 12.0g, Total Carbs: 3.8g, Sugars: 2.2g, Protein:14.1g

66. Rice Pudding

Preparation Time: 5 minutes - **Cooking Time**: 15 minutes - **Servings:** 5

- 1 cup of brown rice
- 2 cups coconut milk, unsweetened
- 1 teaspoon cinnamon
- 1 teaspoon ginger
- 1/3 teaspoon thyme
- 1/3 cup almonds
- 2 tablespoon honey
- 1 teaspoon lemon zest

1. Pour the coconut milk into a saucepan and heat until low.
2. Add the brown rice and stir the mixture carefully.
3. Close the lid and cook the brown rice over medium heat for 10 minutes.
4. Meanwhile, crush the almonds and combine them with the lemon zest, thyme, ginger, and cinnamon.
5. Sprinkle the brown rice with the almond mixture and stir it carefully.
6. Close the lid and cook the dish for 5 minutes.
7. Remove it from the saucepan when the pudding is cooked, and transfer it to a large bowl.
8. Add the honey and stir the pudding.
9. Serve it immediately.

Nutrition: Calories: 423, Fat: 27.1g, Total Carbs: 43.3g, Sugars: 10.4g, Protein: 6.5g

67. Creamy Millet

Preparation Time: 10 minutes - **Cooking Time:** 15 minutes - **Servings:** 8

- 2 cups millet
- 1 cup almond milk, unsweetened
- 1 cup of water
- 1 cup coconut milk, unsweetened
- 1 teaspoon cinnamon
- ½ teaspoon ground ginger
- ¼ teaspoon salt
- 1 tablespoon chia seeds
- 1 tablespoon cashew butter
- 4 oz. Parmesan cheese, grated

1. Combine the coconut milk, almond milk, and water together in the saucepan.
2. Stir the liquid gently and add millet.
3. Mix carefully and close the lid.
4. Cook the millet on the medium heat for 5 minutes.
5. Sprinkle the porridge with the cinnamon, ground ginger, salt, and chia seeds.
6. Carefully stir the mixture with a spoon and proceed to cook for 5 minutes more on medium heat.
7. Add the cashew butter and cook the millet for 5 minutes.
8. Remove the millet from the heat and transfer it to serving bowls.
9. Sprinkle the dish with the grated cheese.

Nutrition: Calories: 384, Fat: 19.8g, Total Carbs: 42.9g, Sugars: 3.6g, Protein: 11.7g

68. Apple Muffins

Preparation Time: 10 minutes - **Cooking Time:** 15 minutes - **Servings:** 5

- 2 eggs
- 1 cup oat flour
- ½ teaspoon salt
- 2 tablespoon stevia
- 3 apples, washed and peeled
- ½ cup skim milk
- 1 tablespoon olive oil
- ½ teaspoon baking soda
- 1 teaspoon apple cider vinegar

1. In the mixing bowl, beat and whisk the eggs well.
2. Add the skim milk, salt, baking soda, stevia, and apple cider vinegar.
3. Stir the mixture carefully.
4. Grate the apples and add the grated mixture in the egg mixture.
5. Stir it carefully and add the oat flour.
6. Add the olive oil and blend into a smooth batter
7. Preheat the oven to 350 F.
8. Fill each muffin from halfway with the batter and place the muffins in the oven.
9. Cook the dish for 15 minutes.
10. Remove the cooked muffins from the oven.
11. Cool the cooked muffins well and serve them.

Nutrition: Calories: 20, Fat: 6.0g, Total Carbs: 32.4g, Sugars: 15.3g, Protein:11.7g

69. Mushroom Frittata

Preparation Time: 10 minutes - **Cooking Time:** 20 minutes - **Servings:** 5

- 8 oz. shiitake mushrooms
- 1 teaspoon salt
- 1 cup broccoli
- 7 eggs
- 5 oz. Parmesan cheese
- 1 tablespoon olive oil
- ½ teaspoon ground ginger
- 5 garlic cloves
- 1 teaspoon oregano
- 1 teaspoon basil
- 1 teaspoon cilantro
- ½cuplow-
- Fat milk

1. Wash the shiitake mushrooms well and chop them.
2. Chop the broccoli and combine it with the mushrooms in a mixing bowl.
3. In a separate bowl, beat the eggs.
4. Sprinkle the egg mixture with the cilantro, basil, oregano, and ground ginger. Stir it well.
5. Add the low-Fat milk and broccoli. Stir the egg mixture well.
6. Peel the garlic cloves and mince them.
7. Add minced garlic in the egg mixture and stir it gently.
8. Preheat the oven to 350 F.
9. Spray a deep pan with olive oil
10. Into the pan, pour the egg mixture and put it in the preheated oven.
11. Cook the frittata for 20 minutes.
12. Remove it from the oven when the dish is baked, and cool slightly.

Nutrition: Calories: 250, Fat: 15.5g, Total Carbs: 11.5g, Sugars: 3.7g, Protein: 19.2g

70. Homemade Granola Bowl

Preparation Time: 10 minutes - **Cooking Time:** 20 minutes - **Servings:** 6

- 3 tablespoons pumpkin seeds
- 1 tablespoon coconut oil
- 1 teaspoon sunflower seeds
- ¼ cup almonds
- 1 cup raw oats
- 3 tablespoons sesame seeds
- 5 tablespoons honey
- 2 cups almond milk, unsweetened

1. Combine the pumpkin seeds, sunflower seeds, almonds, and sesame seeds together.
2. Crush the mixture well and add raw oats.
3. Add the honey and coconut oil.
4. Stir the mixture carefully until you get a smooth mix.
5. Preheat the oven to 350 F.
6. Cover the tray with parchment and transfer the seed mixture onto the tray. Flatten it well.
7. In the preheated oven, bring the tray in and cook for 20 minutes.
8. When the mixture is cooked, remove it from the oven and chill well.
9. Separate the mixture into small pieces and put in serving bowls.
10. Add the almond milk and mix up the dish.

Nutrition: Calories: 381, Fat: 28.5g, Total Carbs: 30.8g, Sugars: 17.4g, Protein: 6.4g

71. Steak with Veggies

Preparation Time: 15 minutes - **Cooking Time:** 12 minutes - **Servings:** 4

- 2 tablespoons coconut oil

- 4 garlic cloves, minced
- 1-pound beef sirloin steak, cut into bite-sized pieces Ground black pepper, as required
- 1½ cups carrots, peeled and cut into matchsticks 1½ cups fresh kale, tough ribs removed and chopped 3 tablespoons tamari

1. Melt the coconut oil in a wok and sauté the garlic over medium heat for approximately 1 minute.
2. Add the beef and black pepper and stir to combine.
3. Increase the heat to medium-high and cook for about 3-4 minutes or until browned from all sides.
4. Add the carrot, kale and tamari and cook for about 4-5 minutes.
5. Remove from the heat and serve hot.
Nutrition: Calories 311 Total Fat 13.8 g Saturated Fat 8.6 g Cholesterol 101 mg Sodium 700 mg Total Carbs 8.4 g Fiber 1.6 g Sugar 2.3 g Protein 37.1 g

72. Shrimp with Veggies

Preparation Time: 15 minutes   - **Cooking Time:** 8 minutes - **Servings:** 5
For Sauce:
- 1 tablespoon fresh ginger, grated
- 2 garlic cloves, minced
- 3 tablespoons low-sodium soy sauce
- 1 tablespoon red wine vinegar
- 1 teaspoon brown sugar
- ¼ teaspoon red pepper flakes, crushed

For Shrimp Mixture:
- 3 tablespoons olive oil
- 1½ pounds medium shrimp, peeled and deveined
- 12 ounces broccoli florets
- 8 ounces, carrot, peeled and sliced

1. For sauce: in a bowl, place all the ingredients and beat until well combined. Set aside.
2. In a large wok, heat oil over medium-high heat and cook the shrimp for about 2 minutes, stirring occasionally.
3. Add the broccoli and carrot and cook about 3-4 minutes, stirring frequently.
4. Stir in the sauce mixture and cook for about 1-2 minutes.
Nutrition: Calories 298 Total Fat 10.7 g Saturated Fat 1.3 g Cholesterol 305 mg Sodium 882 mg Total Carbs 7 g Fiber 2g Sugar 2.4 g Protein 45.5 g

73. Chickpeas with Swiss Chard

Preparation Time: 15 minutes   - **Cooking Time:** 12 minutes - **Servings:** 4
- 2 tablespoon olive oil
- 2 garlic cloves, sliced thinly
- 1 large tomato, chopped finely
- 2 bunches fresh Swiss chard, trimmed
- 1 (18-ounce) can chickpeas, drained and rinsed
- Salt and ground black pepper, as required
- ¼ cup of water
- 1 tablespoon fresh lemon juice
- 2 tablespoons fresh parsley, chopped

1. Heat the oil in a large nonstick wok over medium heat and sauté the garlic for about 1 minute.
2. Add the tomato and cook for about 2-3 minutes, crushing with the back of the spoon.
3. Stir in remaining ingredients except for the lemon juice and parsley and cook for about 5-7 minutes.
4. Drizzle with the lemon juice and remove from the heat.
5. Serve hot with the garnishing of parsley.

Nutrition: Calories 217 Total Fat 8.3 g Saturated Fat 1 g Cholesterol 0 mg Sodium 171 mg Total Carbs 26.2 g Fiber 6.6 g Sugar 1.8 g Protein 8.8 g

74. Buckwheat Noodles with Chicken

Preparation Time: 20 minutes - **Cooking Time:** 25 minutes - **Servings:** 2
- ½ cup broccoli florets
- ½ cup fresh green beans, trimmed and sliced
- 1 cup fresh kale, tough ribs removed and chopped
- 5 ounces buckwheat noodles
- 1 tablespoon coconut oil
- 1 red onion, chopped finely
- 1 (6-ounce) boneless, skinless chicken breast, cubed
- 2 garlic cloves, chopped finely
- 3 tablespoons low-sodium soy sauce

1. In a medium pan of the boiling water, add the broccoli and green beans and cook for about 4-5 minutes.
2. Add the kale and cook for about 1-2 minutes.
3. Drain the vegetables and transfer into a large bowl. Set aside.
4. In another pan of the lightly salted boiling water, cook the soba noodles for about 5 minutes.
5. Drain the noodles well and then, rinse under cold running water. Set aside.
6. Meanwhile, in a large wok, melt the coconut oil over medium heat and sauté the onion for about 2-3 minutes.
7. Add the cubes of chicken and cook for approximately 5-6 minutes.
8. Add the garlic, soy sauce and a little splash of water and cook for about 2-3 minutes, stirring frequently.
9. Add the cooked vegetables and noodles and cook for about 1-2 minutes, tossing frequently.
10. Serve hot with the garnishing of sesame seeds.
Nutrition: Calories 463 Total Fat 11.7 g Saturated Fat 5.9 g Cholesterol 54 mg Sodium 1000 mg Total Carbs 58.9 g Fiber 7.1 g Sugar 4.6 g Protein 22.5 g

75. Spicy Sesame & Edamame Noodles

Preparation Time: 5 minutes - **Cooking Time:** 15 minutes - **Servings:** 2
- 100 g Blue Dragon Whole-wheat Noodles
- 100 g vegetable 'noodles'
- 2 tbsp. groundnut or coconut oil
- 2 shallots, peeled and finely sliced
- 2 tsp. 'lazy' garlic
- 2 tsp. ginger puree
- 1 red chili, sliced
- 3 tbsp. sesame seeds
- 100 g edamame beans, podded
- 2 tbsp. sesame oil
- 2 tbsp. Blue Dragon soy sauce
- Handful fresh coriander, roughly chopped
- Juice of 1 lime

1. For 4 minutes, boil the noodles, then drain and set aside. Cook the vegetable noodles according to the Directions: and add the rest of the noodles.
2. In a big pan or kettle heat the oil and add garlic, ginger and pepper. Cook for 2 minutes and then add sesame seeds and bean sprouts. Cook for another 2 minutes, stir and stir to make sure nothing sticks to the bottom of the pot.
3. Pour the noodles and the noodles into the pan and cook for 2 minutes.

4. Turn off the heat, then add sesame oil, soy sauce and lemon juice and mix. Serve with scattered coriander.
Nutrition: Calories 230 Carbs 25g Fat 13g Protein 4g

76. *Triple Berry Millet Bake*

This breakfast bake is full of blueberries, raspberries, and strawberries, which are then complemented with walnuts? Enjoy it alone or with shavings of dark chocolate over the top.
kilocalories Per Individual Serving: 342
The Number of Servings: 8
Time to prepare/Cook: 70 minutes
- Millet - 1.5 cups
- Soy milk, unsweetened - 2 cups
- Water - 1 cup
- Date sugar - .5 cup
- Vanilla extract - 2 teaspoons
- Sea salt - .25 teaspoon
- Cinnamon - .5 teaspoon
- Walnuts, chopped - 1 cup
- Blueberries, thawed if frozen - 12 ounces
- Strawberries, sliced, thawed if frozen - 8 ounces
- Raspberries, thawed if frozen - 8 ounces

1. Set your oven to Fahrenheit three-hundred and seventy-five degrees and prepare a glass 9-inch by thirteen-inch baking dish.
2. In a large kitchen bowl, whisk together the soy milk, water, millet, date sugar, cinnamon, sea salt, and vanilla extract. Pour the mixture into the prepared pan.
3. Sprinkle the berries and almonds evenly over the top of the pan, and then use a spatula or spoon to slightly press the nuts down into the mixture.
4. Bake the millet until hot and bubbling, about one hour. Remove the millet bake from the oven and allow it to sit for fifteen minutes before serving.

77. *Green Shakshuka*

This shakshuka is a twist on the original, with kale, zucchini, Brussels sprouts, and more, to give you a filling and healthy start to your day.
kilocalories Per Individual Serving: 364
The Number of Servings: 3
Time to Prepare/Cook: 17 minutes
- Zucchini, grated - 1
- Brussels sprouts, finely sliced or shaved - 9 ounces
- Red onion, diced - 1
- Olive oil - 2 tablespoons
- Eggs - 5
- Parsley, chopped - .25 cup
- Kale, chopped - 2 cups
- Sea salt - .5 teaspoon
- Cumin - 1 teaspoon
- Avocado, sliced - 1

1. In large steel, the skillet salutes the red onion in the olive oil until it becomes slightly transparent, about three minutes. Add in the minced garlic and cook the onion/garlic mixture for an additional minute.
2. Add the Brussels sprouts to the skillet containing the onion and garlic, and cook it for four to five minutes until softened, stirring frequently. Stir in the spices and zucchini, cooking for an additional minute.
3. Stir the kale into the skillet and continue to stir until it begins to wilt. Reduce the heat to low.

4. Using a spatula flatten the shakshuka mixture in the skillet and create five small wells for the eggs to next in. Crack an egg into each of the shakshuka wells and cover the skillet with a lid to steam the eggs until they fit your liking.
5. Top the dish off with the parsley and avocado, serving immediately.

78. *Kale and Butternut Bowls*

You can easily make the vegetable portion of this dish ahead of time and store it in the fridge or freezer. This will encourage you to reheat it in the mornings easily and serve it with little effort alongside an egg.
kilocalories Per Individual Serving: 324
The Number of Servings: 4
Time to Prepare/Cook: 60 minutes
- Red onion, diced - 1
- Butternut squash, seeds removed and cut into quarters - 1
- Kale, chopped - 3 cups
- Garlic, minced - 2 cloves
- Extra virgin olive oil - 1 tablespoon
- Oregano, dried - 1 teaspoon
- Cinnamon - .25 teaspoon
- Turmeric powder - .5 teaspoon
- Sea salt - 1 teaspoon
- Avocado, sliced - 1
- Eggs - 4
- Parsley, chopped - .25 cup
- Black pepper, ground - .25 teaspoon

1. Set the oven to Fahrenheit four-hundred and twenty-five degrees. Place the butternut squash on a pan upside-down so that the skin side is facing upward. Roast the butternut squash until it is fork-tender, about twenty-five to thirty minutes.
2. Allow the butternut squash to cool enough to handle easily, and then peel the skin off with your hands. Slice the butternut squash into bite-size cubes.
3. Heat the extra virgin olive oil in a large skillet over medium heat and saute the onion for about five minutes until it is translucent. Add in the kale, garlic, and seasonings, cooking until the kale is wilted. Add in the butternut squash.
4. Divide the skillet mixture between four serving bowls and top each one with an egg cooked to your choice, sliced avocado, and parsley.

79. *Egg Casserole*

This casserole is full of flavor from your favorite breakfast sausage, vegetables and fresh herbs. You can easily make this at the beginning of the week, and then store it in the fridge for a quick and easy go-to meal.
kilocalories Per Individual Serving: 309
The Number of Servings: 6
Time to Prepare/Cook: 40 minutes
- Eggs - 10
- Breakfast sausage - 1 pound
- Button mushrooms, sliced - 2 cups
- Roma tomatoes, seeded and diced - 3
- Red onion, thinly sliced - 1
- Kale, chopped - 2 cups
- Basil, chopped - 1 tablespoon
- Parsley, chopped - 2 tablespoons
- Sea salt - 1.5 teaspoons

1. Set your oven to Fahrenheit three-hundred and fifty degrees and prepare a nine-inch by thirteen-inch baking dish.
2. In a skillet over medium-high brown, your breakfast sausage until fully cooked, draining off any excess fat.
3. Into the skillet with the breakfast sausage, add the mushrooms, allowing them to saute until tender, about five to seven minutes. Add in the sea salt and remaining vegetables, cooking for an additional two to three minutes until just slightly tender.
4. Transfer the vegetable sausage mixture to the prepared pan.
5. Whisk together the eggs in a large bowl, ensuring the whites fully break down into the yolks. Pour the eggs over the breakfast sausage and mix vegetables, then placing it in the oven to roast until cooked through, about twenty-five to thirty minutes.

80. Vegan Tofu Omelet

This vegan omelet uses tofu to create an egg-like texture, and black salt to give it an egg-like flavor. You can buy black salt online and at specialty stores. If you can't find black salt, you can replace it with regular sea salt, but know it won't have the same egg-like flavor.

kilocalories Per Individual Serving: 276
The Number of Servings: 1
Time to Prepare/Cook: 15 minutes

- Silken tofu - 6 ounces Tahini - 1 teaspoon (optional)
- Cornstarch - 1 tablespoon
- Nutritional yeast - 1 tablespoon
- Soy milk, unsweetened - 1 tablespoon
- Turmeric, ground - .125 teaspoon
- Onion powder - .25 teaspoon
- Sea salt - .25 teaspoon
- Smoked paprika - .125 teaspoon (optional)
- Black salt - .25 teaspoon
- Kale, chopped - .5 cup
- Button mushrooms, sliced - .25 cup
- Onion, diced - 2 tablespoons
- Garlic, minced - 1 clove
- Extra virgin olive oil - 1 tablespoon, dived

1. Into a blender, add the tofu, tahini, cornstarch, yeast, soy milk, turmeric, onion powder, smoked paprika, and bath salts.Pulse on high until fully blended with the mixture.
2. In a skillet, add half of the olive oil along with the vegetables and garlic. Saute until they become tender, about five minutes over medium heat.
3. Meanwhile, add the remaining half of the olive oil to a non-stick medium skillet over medium-high heat. Allow this skillet to preheat while you cook the vegetables until it is very hot. Once hot, pour the tofu batter into the skillet, slightly tilting the pan so that the egg forms a circular shape. You can use a spoon to smooth out the top.
4. Sprinkle the cooked vegetables over the tofu "egg" and reduce the heat of the skillet to medium-low. Cover the skillet with a lid, allowing it to cook three to five minutes until the tofu "egg" is set and the edges have dried. You can use a spatula to lightly lift the edges of the omelet and ensure it is fully set. The coloring should be golden with some browned spots.
5. When ready, loosen the omelet by lifting it with the spatula and then flip one side over the other. Transfer the tofu omelet to a plate and enjoy while warm.

81. Grapefruit & Celery Blast

- 1 grapefruit, peeled
- 2 stalks of celery
- 50g (2oz) kale
- ½ teaspoon matcha powder

The Number of Servings: 1, 71 calories per serving
1. Place all the ingredients into a blender with enough water to cover them and blitz until smooth.

82. Orange & Celery Crush

- 1 carrot, peeled
- 3 stalks of celery
- 1 orange, peeled
- ½ teaspoon matcha powder
- Juice of 1 lime

The Number of Servings: 1, 95 calories per serving
1. Place all of the ingredients into a blender with enough water to cover them and blitz until smooth.

83. Tropical Chocolate Delight

- 1 mango, peeled & de-stoned
- 75g (3oz) fresh pineapple, chopped
- 50g (2oz) kale
- 25g (1oz) rocket
- 1 tablespoon 100% cocoa powder or cacao nibs 150mls (5fl oz) coconut milk

The Number of Servings: 1, 427 calories per serving
1. Place all of the ingredients into a blender and blitz until smooth. When it seems too thick, you should add a little water.

84. Walnut & Spiced Apple Tonic

- 6 walnuts halves
- 1 apple, cored
- 1 banana
- ½ teaspoon matcha powder
- ½ teaspoon cinnamon
- Pinch of ground nutmeg

The Number of Servings: 1, 272 calories per serving
1. Place all of the ingredients into a blender and add sufficient water to cover them. Blitz until smooth and creamy.

85. Sweet Rocket (Arugula) Boost

- 25g (1oz) fresh rocket (arugula) leaves
- 75g (3oz) kale
- 1 apple
- 1 carrot
- 1 tablespoon fresh parsley
- Juice of 1 lime

The Number of Servings: 1, 113 calories per serving
1. Place all of the ingredients into a blender with enough water to cover and process until smooth.

86. Banana & Ginger Snap

- 2.5cm (1 inch) chunk of fresh ginger, peeled
- 1 banana
- 1 large carrot
- 1 apple, cored
- ½ stick of celery
- ¼ level teaspoon turmeric powder

The Number of Servings: 1, 166 calories per serving
1. Place all the ingredients into a blender with just enough water to cover them.
2. Process until smooth

87. Chocolate, Strawberry & Coconut Crush
- 100mls (3½fl oz) coconut milk
- 100g (3½oz) strawberries
- 1 banana
- 1 tablespoon 100% cocoa powder or cacao nibs
- 1 teaspoon matcha powder

The Number of Servings: 1, 324 calories per serving
1. Toss all of the ingredients into a blender and process them to a creamy consistency. Add a little additional water if you need to thin it out a little.
2.

88. Chocolate Berry Blend
- 50g (2oz) kale
- 50g (2oz) blueberries
- 50g (2oz) strawberries
- 1 banana
- 1 tablespoon 100% cocoa powder or cacao nibs 200mls (7fl oz) unsweetened soya milk

The Number of Servings: 1, 241 calories per serving

1. Place all of the ingredients into a blender with enough water to cover them and process until smooth.

89. Cranberry & Kale Crush
- 75g (3oz) strawberries
- 50g (2oz) kale
- 120mls (4fl oz) unsweetened cranberry juice 1 teaspoon chia seeds
- ½ teaspoon matcha powder

The Number of Servings: 1, 71 calories per serving
1. Place all of the ingredients into a blender and process until smooth. Add some crushed ice and a mint leaf or two for a refreshing drink.

90. Poached Eggs & Rocket (Arugula)
- 2 eggs
- 25g (1oz) fresh rocket (arugula)
- 1 teaspoon olive oil
- Sea salt
- Freshly ground black pepper

The Number of Servings: 1, 178 calories per serving
1. Scatter the rocket (arugula) leaves onto a plate and drizzle the olive oil over them. Bring a shallow pan of water to the boil, Put the eggs in and cook until the whites are strong. Serve the eggs on top of the rocket and season with salt and pepper.

91. Strawberry Buckwheat Pancakes
- 100g (3½oz) strawberries, chopped
- 100g (3½ oz) buckwheat flour
- 1 egg
- 250mls (8fl oz) milk
- 1 teaspoon olive oil
- 1 teaspoon olive oil for frying

- Freshly squeezed juice of 1 orange

The Number of Servings: 4, 175 calories per serving
1. Pour the milk into a bowl and mix in the egg and a teaspoon of olive oil. Sift in the flour to the liquid mixture until smooth and creamy. Allow it to rest for 15 minutes. Heat a little oil in a pan and pour in a quarter of the mixture (or to the size you prefer.) Sprinkle in a quarter of the strawberries into the batter—Cook for around 2 minutes on each side. Serve hot with a drizzle of orange juice. You could try experimenting with other berries such as blueberries and blackberries.

92. Strawberry & Nut Granola
- 200g (7oz) oats
- 250g (9oz) buckwheat flakes
- 100g (3½ oz) walnuts, chopped
- 100g (3½ oz) almonds, chopped
- 100g (3½ oz) dried strawberries
- 1½ teaspoons ground ginger
- 1½ teaspoons ground cinnamon
- 120mls (4fl oz) olive oil
- 2 tablespoon honey

The Number of Servings: 12, 391 calories per serving
1. Combine the oats, buckwheat flakes, nuts, ginger and cinnamon. In a saucepan, warm the oil and honey,. Stir until the honey has melted. Pour the warm oil into the dry ingredients and mix well. Spread the mixture out on a large baking tray (or two) and bake in the oven at 150C (300F) for around 50 minutes until the granola is golden. Allow it to cool. Add in the dried berries. Store in an airtight container until ready to use. Can be served with yogurt, milk or even dry as a handy snack.

93. Chilled Strawberry & Walnut Porridge
- 100g (3½ oz) strawberries
- 50g (2oz) rolled oats
- 4 walnut halves, chopped
- 1 teaspoon chia seeds
- 200mls (7fl oz) unsweetened soya milk 100ml (3½ fl oz) water

The Number of Servings: 1, 384 calories
1. Place the strawberries, oats, soya milk and water into a blender and process until smooth. Stir in the chia seeds and mix well. Chill in the fridge overnight and serve in the morning with a sprinkling of chopped walnuts. It's simple and delicious.

94. Fruit & Nut Yogurt Crunch
- 100g (3½ oz) plain Greek yogurt
- 50g (2oz) strawberries, chopped
- 6 walnut halves, chopped
- The sprinkling of cocoa powder

The Number of Servings: 1, 296 calories
1. Stir half of the chopped strawberries into the yogurt. Using a glass, place a layer of yogurt with a sprinkling of strawberries and walnuts, followed by another layer of the same until you reach the top of the glass.
2. Garnish with walnuts pieces and a dusting of cocoa powder.

95. Cheesy Baked Eggs
- 4 large eggs
- 75g (3oz) cheese, grated

- 25g (1oz) fresh rocket (arugula) leaves, finely chopped
- 1 tablespoon parsley
- ½ teaspoon ground turmeric
- 1 tablespoon olive oil

The Number of Servings: 4, 198 calories per serving

1. Grease each ramekin dish with a little olive oil. Divide the rocket (arugula) between the ramekin dishes then break an egg into each one. Sprinkle a little parsley and turmeric on top then sprinkle on the cheese. In a preheated oven, place the ramekins at220C/425F for 15 minutes, until the eggs are set and the cheese is bubbling.

96. Spiced Scramble

- 25g (1oz) kale, finely chopped
- 2 eggs
- 1 spring onion (scallion) finely chopped
- 1 teaspoon turmeric
- 1 tablespoon olive oil
- Sea salt

Freshly ground black pepper 259 calories per serving

The Number of Servings: 1

1. Crack the eggs into a bowl. Add the turmeric and whisk them— season with salt and pepper. Heat the oil in a frying pan, add the kale and spring onions (scallions) and cook until it has wilted. Pour in the beaten eggs and stir until eggs have scrambled together with the kale.

97. Sirtfood Mushroom Scramble Eggs

- 2 tbsp.
- 1 teaspoon ground garlic
- 1 teaspoon mild curry powder
- 20g lettuce, approximately sliced
- 1 teaspoon extra virgin olive oil
- 1/2 bird's eye peeled, thinly chopped
- A couple of mushrooms, finely chopped 5g parsley, finely chopped
- *elective * insert a seed mix for a topper plus some rooster sauce for taste

1. Mix the curry and garlic powder and then add just a little water till you've achieved a light glue.
2. Steam the lettuce for two -- 3 minutes.
3. Eat the oil over a moderate heat in a skillet and fry the chili and mushrooms 2-3 minutes till they've begun to soften and brown.
4. Insert the eggs and spice paste and cook over moderate heat, then add the carrot and then proceed to cook over a moderate heat for a further minute. In the end, put in the parsley, mix well, and function.

98. Blue Hawaii Smoothie

- 2 tablespoons ring or approximately 4-5 balls 1/2 cup frozen tomatoes
- Two tbsp ground flaxseed
- ⅛ cup tender coconut (unsweetened, organic)
- Few walnuts
- 1/2 cup fat-free yogurt
- 5-6 ice cubes Dab of water

1. Throw all of the ingredients together and combine until smooth. You might need to prevent and wake up to receive it combined smoothie or put in more water.

99. Turkey Breakfast Sausages

- 1 lb. extra lean ground turkey
- 1 tbsp. EVOO, and a little more to dirt pan
- 1 tbsp. fennel seeds
- 1 teaspoon smoked paprika
- 1 teaspoon red pepper flakes
- 1 teaspoon peppermint
- 1 teaspoon chicken seasoning
- A couple of shredded cheddar cheese
- A couple of chives, finely chopped
- A few shakes garlic and onion powder
- Two spins of pepper and salt

1. Preheat to 350f.
2. Utilize a little EVOO to dirt a miniature muffin pan.
3. Combine all ingredients and blend thoroughly.
4. Fill each pit on top of the pan and then cook for approximately 15-20 minutes. Each toaster differs; therefore, when muffin fever is 165, then remove.

100. Banana Pecan Muffins

- 3 tbsp. butter softened
- 3 ripe bananas
- 1 tbsp. honey
- ⅛ cup oj
- 1 teaspoon cinnamon
- 1 cups all-purpose pasta
- 2 capsules
- A couple of pecans, sliced
- 1 tbsp. vanilla

1. Preheat the oven to 180°c/ / 350°f.
2. Lightly grease the muffin tin's bottom and sides, and then dust with flour.
3. Dust the surfaces of the tin gently with flour then tap to eradicate any excess.
4. Peel and insert the batter to a mixing bowl and with a fork, mash the carrots; therefore that you've got a combination of chunky and smooth, then put aside.
5. Insert the orange juice, melted butter, eggs, vanilla, and spices and stir to combine.
6. Roughly chop the pecans onto a chopping board, when using, then fold throughout the mix.
7. Spoon at the batter 3/4 full and bake in the oven for approximately 40 minutes, or until golden and cooked through.

Lunch

101. Sticky Chicken Watermelon Noodle Salad

Preparation Time: 20 minutes - **Cooking time:** 40 minutes - **Servings:** 2

- 2 pieces of skinny rice noodles
- 1/2 tbsp. sesame oil
- 2 cups watermelon
- Head of bib lettuce
- Half of a lot of scallions
- Half of a lot of fresh cilantro
- 2 skinless, boneless chicken breasts
- 1/2 tbsp. Chinese five-spice

- 1 tbsp. extra virgin olive oil
- Two tbsp. sweet skillet (I utilized a mixture of maple syrup using a dash of tabasco)
- 1 tbsp. sesame seeds
- A couple of cashews - smashed Dressing - could be made daily or 2 until 1 tbsp. low-salt soy sauce 1 teaspoon sesame oil
- 1 tbsp. peanut butter
- Half of a refreshing red chili
- Half of a couple of chives
- Half of a couple of cilantros
- 1 lime - juiced
- 1 small spoonful of garlic

1. In a bowl, then completely substituting the noodles in boiling drinking water. They are going to be soon spread out in 2 minutes.
2. On a big sheet of parchment paper, throw the chicken with pepper, salt, and the five-spice.
3. Twist over the paper subsequently flattens the chicken using a rolling pin.
4. Place into the large skillet with 1 tbsp. of olive oil, turning 3 or 4 minutes, until well charred and cooked through.
5. Using 1 tbsp to remove the noodles and toss. Sesame oil on a large serving platter.
6. Place 50% the noodles into the moderate skillet, frequently stirring until crispy and nice.
7. Remove the watermelon skin, then slice the flesh to inconsistent balls, and then move to plate.
8. Wash the lettuces and cut into small wedges and half of a whole lot of leafy greens and scatter on the dish.
9. Place another 1 / 2 the cilantro pack, the soy sauce, coriander, chives, peanut butter, 1 teaspoon of sesame oil, a dab of water, and the lime juice in a bowl, then mix till smooth.
10. set the chicken back to heat, garnish with all the sweet sauce (or my walnut syrup mixture) and toss with the sesame seeds.
11. Pour the dressing on the salad toss gently with clean fingers until well coated, then add crispy noodles and then smashed cashews.
12. Mix chicken pieces and add them to the salad.
Nutrition: Calories: 694 Carbohydrates: 0 Fat: 33g Protein: 0

102. Fruity Curry Chicken Salad

Preparation Time: 20 minutes - **Cooking time:** 10 minutes - **Servings:** 2
- Original recipe yields 8 servings
- Fixing checklist
- 4 skinless, boneless chicken pliers - cooked and diced
- 1 tsp celery, diced
- 4 green onions, sliced
- 1 golden delicious apple peeled, cored, and diced
- 1/3 cup golden raisins
- 1/3 cup seedless green grapes, halved
- 1/2 cup sliced toasted pecans
- 1/8 Teaspoon ground black pepper
- 1/2 tsp curry powder
- 3/4 cup light mayonnaise

1. In a big bowl, combine the chicken, onion, celery, apple, celery, celery, pecans, pepper, curry powder, and carrot. Mix altogether. Enjoy!

Nutrition: Fat; 44 milligrams Cholesterol: 188 milligrams Sodium. 12.3 g Carbohydrates: 15.1 gram of Protein; full nutrition

103. Zuppa Toscana

Preparation Time: 25 minutes - **Cooking time:** 60 minutes - **Servings**: 2
- 1 lb. ground Italian sausage
- 1 1/4 tsp of crushed of red pepper flakes
- 4 pieces bacon, cut into ½ inch bits
- 1 big onion, diced
- 1 tbsp. minced garlic
- 5 (13.75 oz.) can chicken broth
- 6 celery, thinly chopped
- 1 cup thick cream
- 1/4 bunch fresh spinach, tough stems removed

1. Cook that the Italian sausage and red pepper flakes in a pot on medium-high heat until crumbly, browned, with no longer pink, 10 to 15minutes. Drain and put aside.
2. Cook the bacon at the exact Dutch oven over moderate heat until crispy, about 10 minutes. Drain, leaving a couple of tablespoons of drippings together with all the bacon at the bottom of the toaster. Stir in the garlic and onions cook until onions are tender and translucent, about five minutes.
3. Pour the chicken broth to the pot with the onion and bacon mix; contribute to a boil on high temperature. Add the berries and boil until fork-tender, about 20 minutes.
4. Reduce heat to moderate and stir in the cream and the cooked sausage – heat throughout. Mix the lettuce to the soup before serving.
Nutrition: Carbohydrates; 32.6 g Fat; 45.8 g Carbs; 19.8 g Protein; 99 Milligrams Cholesterol: 2386

104. Country Chicken Breasts

Preparation Time: 10 minutes - **Cooking Time**: 45 minutes - **Servings**: 2
- 2 medium green apples, diced
- 1 small red onion, finely diced
- 1 small green bell pepper, chopped
- 3 cloves garlic, minced
- 2 tablespoons dried currants
- 1 tablespoon curry powder
- 1 teaspoon turmeric
- 1 teaspoon ground ginger
- ¼ teaspoon chili pepper flakes
- 1 can (14 ½ ounce) diced tomatoes
- 6 skinless, boneless chicken breasts, halved
- ½ cup chicken broth
- 1 cup long-grain white rice
- 1-pound large raw shrimp, shelled and deveined
- Salt and pepper to taste
- Chopped parsley
- 1/3 cup slivered almonds

1. Rinse chicken, pat dry and set aside.
2. In a large crockpot, combine apples, onion, bell pepper, garlic, currants, curry powder, turmeric, ginger, and chili pepper flakes. Stir in tomatoes.
3. Arrange chicken, overlapping pieces slightly, on top of tomato mixture.
4. Pour in broth and do not mix or stir.
5. Cover and cook at for 6 – 7 hours on low.
6. Preheat oven to 200 degrees F.

7. Carefully transfer chicken to an oven-safe plate, cover lightly, and keep warm in the oven.

8. Stir rice into remaining liquid. Increase the heat setting of the cooker to high; cover and cook, stirring once or twice, until rice is almost tender to bite, 30 to 35 minutes. Stir in the shrimp, cover and cook until the middle of the shrimp is opaque,about 10 more minutes.

9. Meanwhile, toast almonds in a small pan over medium heat until golden brown, 5 - 8 minutes, stirring occasionally. Set aside.

10. Mound in a warm serving dish and arrange chicken on top. Sprinkle with parsley and almonds.

Nutrition: Calories: 155 Carbs: 13.9g Protein: 17.4g Fat: 3.8g

105. *Apples and Cabbage Mix*

Preparation Time: 5 minutes - **Cooking Time:** 0 minutes - **Servings:** 4

- 2 cored and cubed green apples
- 2tbsps. Balsamic vinegar
- ½ tsp. caraway seeds
- 2tbsps. olive oil
- Black pepper
- 1 shredded red cabbage head

1. Mix the cabbage with the apples and the other ingredients in a dish, toss and serve.

Nutrition: Calories: 165 Fat: 7.4 g Carbs: 26 g Protein: 2.6 g Sugars: 2.6 g Sodium: 19 mg

106. *Rosemary Endives*

Preparation Time: 10 minutes - **Cooking Time:** 45 minutes - **Servings:** 2

- 2tbsps. olive oil
- 1 tsp. dried rosemary
- 2 halved endives
- ¼ tsp. black pepper
- ½ tsp. turmeric powder

1. In a baking pan, combine the endives with the oil and the other ingredients, toss gently, introduce in the oven and bake at 400 0F for 20 minutes.

2. Divide between plates and serve.

Nutrition: Calories: 66 Fat: 7.1 g Carbs: 1.2 g Protein: 0.3 g Sugars: 1.3 g Sodium: 113 mg

107. *Kale Sauté*

Preparation Time: 10 minutes - **Cooking Time:** 35 minutes - **Servings:** 2

- 1 chopped red onion
- 3tbsps. coconut aminos
- 2tbsps. olive oil
- 1 lb. torn kale
- 1 tbsp. chopped cilantro
- 1 tbsp. lime juice
- 2 minced garlic cloves

1. Heat a pan over medium heat with the olive oil, add the onion and the garlic and sauté for 5 minutes.

2. Add the kale and the other ingredients, toss, cook over medium heat for 10 minutes, divide between plates and serve.

Nutrition: Calories: 200 Fat: 7.1 g Carbs: 6.4 g Protein: 6 g Sugars: 1.6 g Sodium: 183 mg

108. *Roasted Beets*

Preparation Time: 10 minutes - **Cooking Time:** 40 minutes - **Servings:** 2

- 2 minced garlic cloves
- ¼ tsp. black pepper
- 4 peeled and sliced beets
- ¼ c. chopped walnuts
- 2tbsps. olive oil
- ¼ c. chopped parsley

1. In a baking dish, combine the beets with the oil and the other ingredients, toss to coat, introduce in the oven at 420 0F, and bake for 30 minutes.

2. Divide between plates and serve.

Nutrition: Calories: 156 Fat: 11.8 g Carbs: 11.5 g Protein: 3.8 g Sugars: 8 g Sodium: 670 mg

109. *Minty Tomatoes and Corn*

Preparation Time: 10 minutes - **Cooking Time:** 65 minutes - **Servings:** 2

- 2 c. corn
- 1 tbsp. rosemary vinegar
- 2tbsps. chopped minutest
- 1 lb. sliced tomatoes
- ¼ tsp. black pepper
- 2tbsps. olive oil

1. In a salad bowl, combine the tomatoes with the corn and the other ingredients, toss and serve.

Nutrition: Calories: 230 Fat: 7.2 g Carbs: 11.6 g Protein: 4 g Sugars: 1 g Sodium: 53 mg

110. *Pesto Green Beans*

Preparation Time: 10 minutes - **Cooking Time:** 55 minutes - **Servings:** 2

- 2tbsps. olive oil
- 2 tsps. Sweet paprika
- Juice of 1 lemon
- 2tbsps. basil pesto
- 1 lb. trimmed and halved green beans
- ¼ tsp. black pepper
- 1 sliced red onion
- Over medium-high pressure, heat a pan with the oil, add the onion, stir and sauté for 5 minutes.
- Add the beans and the rest of the ingredients, toss, cook over medium heat for 10 minutes, divide between plates and serve.

Nutrition: Calories: 280 Fat: 10 g Carbs: 13.9 g Protein: 4.7 g Sugars: 0.8 g Sodium: 138 mg

111. *Scallops and Sweet Potatoes*

Preparation Time: 5 minutes - **Cooking Time:** 22 minutes - **Servings:** 4

- 1-pound scallops
- ½ teaspoon rosemary, dried
- ½ teaspoon oregano, dried
- 2 tablespoons avocado oil
- 1 yellow onion, chopped
- 2 sweet potatoes, peeled and cubed
- ½ cup chicken stock
- 1 tablespoon cilantro, chopped

1. Heat a pan with the oil on medium heat, add the onion and sauté for 2 minutes.

2. Add the sweet potatoes and the stock, toss and cook for 10 minutes more.
3. Add the scallops and the remaining ingredients, toss, cook for another10 minutes, divide everything into bowls and serve.
Nutrition: Calories 211 Fat 2 Fiber 4.1 Carbs 26.9 Protein 20.7

112. *Citrus Salmon*

Preparation Time: 10 minutes - **Cooking Time:** 45 minutes - **Servings:** 2
- 1 ½ lb. salmon fillet with skin on
- Salt and pepper to taste
- 1 medium red onion, chopped
- 2 tablespoons parsley, chopped
- 2 teaspoons lemon rind, grated
- 2 teaspoons orange rind, grated
- 2 tablespoons extra virgin olive oil
- 1 lemon, sliced thinly
- 1 orange, sliced thinly
- 1 cup vegetable broth

1. Line your crockpot with parchment paper and top with the lemon slices.
2. Season salmon with salt and pepper and place it on top of lemon.
3. Cover the fish with the onion, parsley and grated citrus rinds and oil over fish. Top with orange slices, reserving a few for garnish.
4. Pour broth around, but not directly overtop, your salmon.
5. Cover and cook for 2 hours under low pressure.
6. Preheat oven to 400 degrees F.
7. When salmon is opaque and flaky, remove from the crockpot carefully using the parchment paper and transfer to a baking sheet. Place in the oven for 5 – 8 minutes to allow the salmon to brown on top.
8. Serve garnished with orange and lemon slices.
Nutrition: Calories 294 Fat 3 Fiber 8 Carbs 49 Protein 21

113. *Sage Carrots*

Preparation Time: 10 minutes - **Cooking Time**: 25 minutes - **Servings:** 2
- 2 tsps. Sweet paprika
- 1 tbsp. chopped sage
- 2tbsps. olive oil
- 1 lb. peeled and roughly cubed carrots
- ¼ tsp. black pepper
- 1 chopped red onion

1. In a baking pan, combine the carrots with the oil and the other ingredients, toss and bake at 380 0F for 30 minutes.
2. Divide between plates and serve.
Nutrition: Calories: 200 Fat: 8.7 g Carbs: 7.9 g Protein: 4 g Sugars: 19 g Sodium: 268 mg

114. *Moong Dahl*

Preparation Time: 10 minutes - **Cooking Time:** 10 minutes - **Servings:** 4-6
- 300g/10oz split mung beans (moong dahl)
- Preferably soaked for a few hours
- 600ml/1pt of water
- 2 tbsp./30g olive oil, butter or ghee
- 1 red onion, finely chopped
- 1-2 tsp coriander seeds
- 1-2 tsp cumin seeds
- 2-4 tsp fresh ginger, chopped
- 1-2 tsp turmeric
- ¼ tsp of cayenne pepper – more if you want it spicy
- Salt & black pepper to taste

1. First drain and rinse the split mung beans. Put them in a saucepan, then cover them with water. Bring to the boil and skim off any foam that arises. Turn down the heat, cover and simmer.
2. Meanwhile, in a pan, heat the oil and fry the onion until the onion becomes soft.
3. In a heavy-bottomed pan, fry the coriander and cumin seeds dryly. Fry until they start to pop. Grind them in a pestle and mortar.
4. Add the ground spices to the onions and also add ginger, turmeric and cayenne pepper. Cook for a few minutes.
5. Once the mung beans are almost done, add the onion and spice mix to them. With salt and pepper, season and cook for another 10 minutes.
Nutrition: Calories 347 Protein 25.73 Fiber 18.06

115. *Macaroni & Cheese with Broccoli*

Preparation Time: 10 minutes - **Cooking Time:** 6 minutes - **Servings**: 6
- 3cups whole-wheat macaroni, uncooked 1large fresh broccoli crown, chopped ¼cup flour
- 2.5cups milk, divided
- 1½cups shredded extra-sharp cheddar cheese 2teaspoons Dijon mustard
- ¼teaspoon garlic powder
- ¾teaspoon paprika
- ¼teaspoon salt
- 2teaspoons extra virgin olive oil
- Crumb topping
- Cooking spray
- 3tablespoons dry breadcrumbs
- ¾teaspoon salt
- ¼teaspoon white pepper

1. Preheat oven to 400° F. Coat a 2-quart baking dish with cooking spray. Bring to a boil a large pot of salted water.
2. When water boils cook macaroni 4 minutes. Add the raw fresh broccoli. Continue to cook until the pasta is slightly undercooked, for 2 minutes longer; the broccoli should be bright green and tender.
3. Meanwhile, prepare the sauce with cheese. Heat 2 cups of milk over medium-high heat in a medium saucepan, stirring frequently until heated. In a medium bowl, whisk together the remaining ½ cup of cold milk, flour, Dijon mustard, ¾ teaspoon salt and white pepper until fully smooth. In the steaming milk, mix the flour mixture and bring to a simmer, whisking frequently until smooth and thickened.
4. In the pasta, stir the cheese sauce. Move the pasta mixture into the baking dish that has been prepared. In a small cup, whisk together the breadcrumbs, paprika, ¼ teaspoon of salt, and garlic powder. Sprinkle with olive oil and stir until completely mixed. The crumbs are poured over the pasta and moved to the oven.
Nutrition: Energy (calories):397; Fat:7.1g; Carbohydrates:59.9g; Protein:20.5g

116. *Glazed Tofu with Vegetables and Buckwheat*

Preparation Time: 10 minutes. - **Cooking Time:** 20 minutes. - **Servings:** 1.
- 150g tofu

- 1 tablespoon of mirin
- 20g Miso paste
- 40g green celery stalk
- 35g red onion
- 120g courgetti
- 1 small Thai chili
- 1 garlic clove
- 1 small piece of ginger
- 50g kale
- 2 teaspoons sesame seeds
- 35g buckwheat
- 1 teaspoon turmeric
- 2 teaspoons of extra virgin olive oil
- 1 teaspoon soy sauce or tamari

1. Preheat oven to 400 °.
2. In the meantime, mix mirin and miso. Cut the tofu in half lengthwise and divide into two triangles. Briefly marinate the tofu with the mirin/miso paste while preparing the other ingredients.
3. Cut the celery stalks into thin slices, the zucchini into thick rings and the onion into thin rings. Finely chop garlic, ginger and chili. Coarsely chop the kale and stew or blanch briefly.
4. Place the marinated tofu in a small casserole dish, sprinkle with the sesame seeds and bake in the oven for approx. 15 minutes until the marinade has caramelized slightly.
5. In the meantime, cook the buckwheat according to the package instructions and add turmeric to the water.
6. Meanwhile, in a coated pan, heat the olive oil and add the celery,, onion, courgette, chili, ginger and garlic—cook over high heat for one to two minutes, then two to three minutes at low temperature. Add a little water as required.
7. Serve the glazed tofu with vegetables and buckwheat.
Nutrition: Calories: 454 Fat: 24.2g. Carbs: 46.5g. Protein: 17.3g.

117. Tofu with Cauliflower
Preparation Time: 10 minutes. - **Cooking Time**: 50 minutes. - **Servings**: 1
- 60g red pepper, seeded
- 1 Thai chili, cut in two halves, seeded
- 2 cloves of garlic
- 1 teaspoon of olive oil
- 1 pinch of cumin
- 1 pinch of coriander
- Juice of a 1/4 lemon
- 200g tofu
- 200g cauliflower, roughly chopped
- 40g red onions, finely chopped
- 1 teaspoon finely chopped ginger
- 2 teaspoons turmeric
- 30g dried tomatoes, finely chopped
- 20g parsley, chopped

1. Preheat oven to 400 °. Slice the peppers and put them in an ovenproof dish with chili and garlic. Pour some olive oil over it, add the dried herbs and put it in the oven Until the softness of the peppers is (about 20 minutes). Let it cool down, put the peppers together with the lemon juice in a blender and work it into a soft mass.
2. Cut the tofu in half and divide the halves into triangles. Place the tofu in a small casserole dish, cover with the paprika mixture and place in the oven for about 20 minutes.
3. Chop the cauliflower until the pieces are smaller than a grain of rice.

4. Then, in a small saucepan, heat the garlic, onions, chili and ginger with olive oil until they become transparent. Add turmeric and cauliflower, mix well and heat again. Remove from heat and add parsley and tomatoes, mix well. Serve with the tofu in the sauce.
Nutrition: Calories: 197.3 Fat: 9.4 g. Carbohydrate: 19.3 g Protein: 13.5 g

118. Filled Pita Pockets
Preparation Time: 20 minutes. - **Cooking Time:** 0 minutes. - **Servings:** 1
- You need whole-grain pita bags.
- For a filling with meat:
- 80g roasted turkey breast
- 25g rocket salad, finely chopped
- 20g cheese, grated
- 35g cucumbers, small diced
- 30g red onions, finely diced
- 15g walnuts, chopped
- Dressing of 1 tablespoon balsamic vinegar and 1 tablespoon extra-virgin olive oil

For a vegan filling:
- 3 tablespoons hummus
- 35g cucumbers, small diced
- 30g red onions, finely diced
- 25g rocket salad, finely chopped
- 15g walnuts, chopped
- Dressing of 1 tablespoon of extra virgin olive oil and some lemon juice

In both variations, mix all the ingredients, fill the pita pockets with them and marinate them with the dressing.
Nutrition: Calories: 120 Fat: 1g. Carbohydrate: 23g. Protein: 21g

119. Lima Bean Dip with Celery and Crackers
Preparation Time: 10 minutes. - **Cooking Time:** 0 minutes. - **Servings:** 2
- 400g Lima beans or white beans from the tin
- 3 tablespoons of olive oil
- Juice and zest of half an untreated lemon
- 4 spring onions, cut into fine rings
- 1 garlic clove, pressed
- 1/4 Thai chili, chopped

1. Drain the beans. Then mix all ingredients with a potato masher to a mass.
2. Serve with green celery sticks and crackers.
Nutrition: Calories: 88 Fat: 0.7g. Carbohydrates: 15.7g. Protein: 5.3g.

120. Spinach and Eggplant Casserole
Preparation Time: 15 minutes. - **Cooking Time:** 55 minutes. - **Servings:** 3
- Eggplant
- Onion slices
- A spoon of olive oil
- 450 g spinach (fresh)
- Tomato
- Egg
- 60 ml of almond milk
- 1 teaspoon lemon juice
- Almond flour

1. Preheat the oven to 200 ° C.
2. Using olive oil to clean the eggplant and onions and fry them in the pan.
3. Place spinach in a large pot, heat over medium heat, then drain the colander.
4. Put the vegetables in a frying pan: first eggplant, then spinach, then onions and tomatoes. Repeat again
5. Beat eggs with almond milk, lemon juice, salt and pepper, then pour them on the vegetables.
6. Sprinkle almond flour on a plate and bake for about 30 to 40 minutes.
Nutrition: Calories: 139.9 Fat: 6.5 g. Carbohydrate: 21.5 g. Protein: 10.3 g.

121. Ancient Mediterranean Pizza

Preparation Time: 45 minutes. - **Cooking Time**: 35 minutes. - **Servings**: 3
- 120 g tapioca flour
- Teaspoon Celtic sea salt
- 1 tablespoon Italian spice mix
- 45 grams of coconut flour
- 120 ml olive oil (fresh) water (hot) 120 ml
- Cover with eggs (slap):
- 1 tablespoon tomato paste (can)
- 1/2 slices zucchini
- 1/2 eggplant
- Tomato slices
- A spoon of olive oil (delicate)
- Balsamic vinegar

1. Preheat the oven to 190 ° C and cover the pan with parchment paper.
2. Cut the vegetables into thin slices.
3. Put cassava flour and salt, Italian herbs and coconut flour together in a large bowl.
4. Pour olive oil and hot water and mix well.
5. Then add the eggs and stir until the dough is even.
6. If it is too thin for the dough, add 1 tablespoon of coconut flour at a time until it reaches the desired thickness. Wait a few minutes before adding more coconut flour, as this will take some time to absorb the water. The purpose is to obtain a soft dough.
7. Divide the dough in half, then wrap it in a circle on the baking sheet (or make a large pizza as shown).
8. Bake for 10 minutes.
9. Brush the pizza with tomato sauce, then sprinkle the eggplant, zucchini and tomatoes on the pizza.
10. Pour the pancakes in olive oil and cook for 10 to15 minutes.
11. Pour balsamic vinegar on pizza before eating.
Nutrition: Calories:221.8 Fat:8.0 Carbs: 31g Protein: 12g

122. Vegetarian Ratatouille

Preparation Time: 20 minutes. - **Cooking Time:** 1 hour. - **Servings:** 1
- 200 grams diced tomatoes (canned)
- 2 slices onion
- Clove garlic
- 4 teaspoons dried oregano
- 4 c. 1 teaspoon paprika
- A spoon of olive oil
- Eggplant
- Zucchini slices
- Pepper
- 1 teaspoon dried thyme

1. Preheat the oven to 180 ° C, then gently lubricate the circle or oval.
2. Finely chop onion and garlic.
3. Mix tomato slices with garlic, onion, oregano and pepper, season with salt and pepper, then put in the bottom of the pot.
4. Use a mandolin, cheese slicer or sharp knife to cut eggplant, zucchini and pepper.
5. Place the vegetables in a bowl (wrapped, starting at the edge and processing inside).
6. Place olive oil on vegetables and sprinkle with thyme, salt and pepper.
7. Cover the pan with parchment paper and bake for 45 to 55 minutes.
Nutrition: Calories: 130 Fat: 1g Carbs: 8g Protein:1g

123. Spicy Spare Ribs with Roasted Pumpkin

Preparation Time: 1 day. - **Cooking Time**: 1 hour and 15 minutes. - **Servings**: 5
- 400g pork ribs
- A spoon of coconut amino acids
- Honey spoon
- A spoon of olive oil
- 50 g shallots
- Garlic clove
- Green paper
- 1 slice onion
- 1 red pepper
- 1 red pepper

For the roasted pumpkin:
- 1 slice of pumpkin
- 1 tablespoon coconut oil
- 1 teaspoon of chili powder

1. Pickled pork ribs the day before yesterday.
2. Cut the ribs into four small pieces: mix coconut amino acids, honey and olive oil in a bowl. Chopped green onions, garlic and peppers, then add. Spread the ribs on the plastic container and pour the marinade. Place them in the refrigerator overnight.
3. Cut onions, peppers and peppers into small pieces and place in a slow cooker. Spare ribs (including marinade) and cook for at least 4 hours.
4. Preheat the pumpkin to 200 ° C.
5. Cut the pumpkin on the moon and place it on a baking sheet lined with parchment paper.
6. Place a spoonful of coconut oil on the baking sheet and season with chili, pepper and salt. Roast the pumpkin in the oven for about 20 minutes, and then serve with the ribs.
Nutrition: Calories: 282 Fat: 18g. Carbs:16g. Protein: 12g.

124. Roast Beef with Grilled Vegetables

Preparation Time: 20 minutes. - **Cooking Time**: 1 hour and 10 minutes. - **Servings**: 5
- 500 g roast beef
- Garlic clove (squeezed)
- One teaspoon fresh rosemary
- 400 g broccoli
- 200g carrots
- 400 g zucchini
- A spoonful of olive oil

1. Rub roast beef with sweet pepper, salt, garlic and rosemary.

2. Heat the pan over high heat and fry the meat for about 20 minutes, Or until, on all sides of the flesh, brown spots emerge. Then wrap it with aluminum foil and let it sit for a while.
3. Then wrap it with aluminum foil and let it sit for a while.
4. Before serving, slice the roast beef into thin slices.
5. Preheat the oven to 205 ° C. Put all the vegetables in the pan.
6. Season the vegetables with a little olive oil and then season with curry and paprika. Bake for 30 minutes or until the vegetables are cooked.
Nutrition: Calories: 347.6 Fat: 8.0g Carbs: 31g Protein: 32.2

125. Turkey meatball skewers

Preparation Time: 5 minutes - **Cooking Time:** 75 minutes - **Servings:** 4
- 4 sticks of lemongrass
- 400g minced turkey
- 2 cloves of garlic, finely chopped
- 1 egg
- 1 red chili, finely chopped
- 2 tablespoons lime juice
- 2 tablespoons chopped coriander
- 1 teaspoon turmeric
- Pepper

1. Clean lemon grass cut in half lengthwise and wash.
2. Mix the meat with the egg, chili, garlic, coriander, olive oil, lime juice, turmeric and a little pepper. Make little balls out of them.
3. Put the balls on the lemongrass skewer and grill them as you like. Cook them in the oven or fry them in the pan until the balls are ready. A small salad goes with it.
Nutrition: Calories 280.0 Fat 35 g Cholesterol 340 mg Fiber 3 g Protein 2.6g

126. Avocado and Cannellini Mash Tacos

Preparation Time: 10 minutes
- 1 ripe avocado, peeled and stoned
- 1 400g can of cannellini beans, drained Juice of 1/2 a lemon
- 1 table spoon olive oil
- Salt and pepper
- A couple of basil leaves
- Taco shells

Place the avocado into a bowl, approximately chop it and then mash it. Consist of the cannellini beans and lemon juice and mash them all together. Stir in the olive oil and season with salt and pepper. Destroy the basil leaves and consist of these.
Fill the taco shells and consume instantly!

127. Almond Butter and Alfalfa Wraps

Preparation Time: 10 minutes
- 4 tablespoon of almond nut butter
- Juice of 1 lemon
- 2-3 carrots-- grated
- 3 radishes, carefully sliced
- 1 cup of alfalfa sprouts
- Salt and pepper
- Lettuce leaves or nori sheets

Mix the almond butter with the majority of the lemon juice and enough water to create a velvety consistency.

Combine the grated carrot, alfalfa sprouts in a bowl. Sprinkle with the remainder of the lemon juice and season with salt and pepper.
Spread the lettuce leaves or nori sheets with almond butter and top with the carrot and grow mixture. Roll up and consume instantly!

128. Asian King Prawn Stir-Fry with Buckwheat Noodles

Preparation time: 10 minutes - Cooking time: 15 minutes
- 150g shelled raw king prawns, deveined
- 2 tea spoon tamari (you can use soy sauce if you are not avoiding gluten)
- 2 tea spoon extra virgin olive oil
- 75g soba (buckwheat noodles)
- 1 garlic clove, finely chopped
- 1 bird's eye chilli, finely chopped
- 1 tea spoon finely chopped fresh ginger
- 20g red onions, sliced
- 40g celery, trimmed and sliced
- 75g green beans, chopped
- 50g kale, roughly chopped
- 100ml chicken stock
- 5g lovage or celery leaves

First heat a frying pan over a high first heat, then cook the prawns in 1 teaspoon of the tamari and 1 teaspoon of the oil for 2–3 minutes. Transfer the prawns to a plate. Wipe the pan out with kitchen paper, as you're going to use it again.
Cook the noodles in boiling water for 5–8 minutes or as directed on the packet. Drain and set aside.
Meanwhile, fry the garlic, chilli and ginger, red onion, celery, beans and kale in the remaining oil over a medium–high first heat for 2–3 minutes. Include the stock and bring to the boil, then simmer for a minute or two, until the vegetables are cooked but still crunchy. Include the prawns, noodles and lovage/celery leaves to the pan, bring back to the boil then remove from the first heat and dish out .

129. Savory Seed Truffles

Preparation time: 10 minutes
- 60g/2oz pumpkin seeds
- 60g/2oz sunflower seeds
- 2 table spoon tahini
- Pinch of cayenne pepper
- Juice of half a lemon
- A handful of coriander leaves
- Salt and pepper

Place the seeds in a food mill with the S blade and grind thoroughly. Include the tahini, cayenne, lemon juice, coriander leaves and salt and pepper.
Process till the mix holds together includeing little quantities of water as r eq uired.
Get rid of the blade from the food mill and form the mix into walnut sized balls.

130. Turmeric Chicken & Kale Salad with Honey Lime Dressing

Preparation time: 20 minutes - Cooking time: 10 minutes
For the chicken
- 1 teaspoon ghee or 1 table spoon coconut oil ½ medium brown onion, diced
- 250-300 g / 9 oz. chicken mince or diced up chicken thighs

- 1 large garlic clove, finely diced
- 1 teaspoon turmeric powder
- 1teaspoon lime zest
- juice of ½ lime
- ½ teaspoon salt + pepper

For the salad
- 6 broccolini stalks or 2 cups of broccoli florets
- 2 tablespoons pumpkin seeds (pepitas)
- 3 large kale leaves, stems removed and chopped
- ½ avocado, sliced
- handful of fresh coriander leaves, chopped handful of fresh parsley leaves, chopped

For the dressing
- 3 tablespoons lime juice
- 1 small garlic clove, finely diced or grated
- 3 tablespoons extra-virgin olive oil (I used 1 tablespoons avocado oil and * 2 tablespoons
- EVO)
- 1 teaspoon raw honey
- ½ teaspoon wholegrain or Dijon mustard
- ½ teaspoon sea salt and pepper

1. First heat the ghee or coconut oil in a small frying pan over medium-high first heat. Include the onion and sauté on medium first heat for 4-5 minutes, until golden. Include the chicken mince and garlic and stir for 2-3 minutes over medium-high first heat, breaking it apart.

2. Include the turmeric, lime zest, lime juice, salt and pepper and cook, stirring frequently, for a further 3-4 minutes. Set the cooked mince aside.

3. While the chicken is cooking, bring a small saucepan of water to boil. Include the broccolini and cook for 2 minutes. Rinse under cold water and cut into 3-4 pieces each.

4. Include the pumpkin seeds to the frying pan from the chicken and toast over medium first heat for 2 minutes, stirring fr eq uently to prevent burning. Season with a little salt. Set aside. Raw pumpkin seeds are also fine to use.

5. Place chopped kale in a salad bowl and pour over the dressing. Using your hands, toss and massage the kale with the dressing. This will soften the kale, kind of like what citrus juice does to fish or beef carpaccio – it 'cooks' it slightly.

6. Finally toss through the cooked chicken, broccolini, fresh herbs, pumpkin seeds and avocado slices.

131. Moong Dahl

Preparation time: 10 minutes - Cooking time: 15 minutes
- 300g/10oz split mung beans (moong dahl)-- preferably soaked for a couple of hours
- 600ml/1pt of water
- 2 table spoon/30g olive butter, oil or ghee
- 1 red onion, finely chopped
- 1-2 tea spoon coriander seeds
- 1-2 tea spoon cumin seeds
- 2-4 tea spoon fresh ginger, sliced
- 1-2 tea spoon turmeric
- If you desire it spicy, 1/4 tea spoon of cayenne pepper--more.
- Salt & black pepper to taste.

Drain and wash the split mung beans. Put them in a pan and cover with the water. Give the boil and skim off any foam that occurs. Decline the very first heat, cover and simmer.
First heat the oil in a pan and sauté the onion till soft.

Dry fry the coriander and cumin seeds in a heavy bottomed pan up until they start to pop. Grind them in a pestle and mortar.
Consist of the ground spices to the onions in addition to the cayenne, turmeric and ginger pepper. Cook for a few minutes.
When the mung beans are almost cooked include the onion and spice mix to them. Season with salt and pepper and cook for an additional 10 minutes.

132. Buckwheat Noodles with Chicken Kale & Miso Dressing

Preparation time: 10 minutes - Cooking time: 15 minutes
For the noodles
- 2-3 handfuls of kale leaves (removed from the stem and roughly cut)
- 150 g / 5 oz buckwheat noodles (100% buckwheat, no wfirst heat)
- 3-4 shiitake mushrooms, sliced
- 1 teaspoon coconut oil or ghee
- 1 brown onion, finely diced
- 1 medium free-range chicken breast, sliced or diced
- 1 long red chilli, thinly sliced (seeds in or out depending on how hot you like it)
- 2 large garlic cloves, finely diced
- 2-3 tablespoons Tamari sauce (gluten-free soy sauce)

For the miso dressing
- 1½ tablespoon fresh organic miso
- 1 tablespoon Tamari sauce
- 1 tablespoon extra-virgin olive oil
- 1 tablespoon lemon or lime juice
- 1 teaspoon sesame oil (optional)

1. Bring a medium saucepan of water to boil. Include the kale and cook for 1 minute, until
slightly wilted. Remove and set aside but reserve the water and bring it back to the boil. Include the soba noodles and cook according to the package steps (usually about 5 minutes). Rinse under cold water and set aside.

2. In the meantime, pan fry the shiitake mushrooms in a little ghee or coconut oil (about a teaspoon) for 2-3 minutes, until lightly browned on each side. Sprinkle with sea salt and set aside.

3. In the same frying pan, first heat more coconut oil or ghee over medium-high first heat. Sauté onion and chilli for 2-3 minutes and then include the chicken pieces. Cook 5 minutes over medium first heat, stirring a couple of times, then include the garlic, tamari sauce and a little splash of water. Cook for a further 2-3 minutes, stirring fr eq uently until chicken is cooked through.

4. Finally, include the kale and soba noodles and toss through the chicken to warm up.

5.Mix the miso dressing and drizzle over the noodles right at the end of cooking, this way you will keep all those beneficial probiotics in the miso alive and active.

133. Courgette Tortilla

Preparation time: 10 minutes - Cooking time: 15 minutes
- 2 table spoon coconut oil or butter
- 1 courgettes, sliced
- 4 eggs, beaten
- A pinch of salt and pepper
- Newly chopped chives or parsley

First heat the oil or butter in a heavy bottomed fry pan and consist of the courgettes. Prepare until soft, stirring sometimes. Mix the salt, pepper, and herbs in with the beaten eggs and consist of to the pan.

Cook till the egg is almost cooked through. End up the cooking by positioning the pan under a medium grill. Dish out with a large green salad.

134. Baked Potatoes with Spicy Chickpea Stew

Preparation time: 10 minutes - Cooking time: 45 minutes
* 4-6 baking potatoes, punctured all over
* 2 tablespoons olive oil
* 2 red onions, finely sliced
* 4 cloves garlic, grated or crushed
* 2cm ginger, grated
* 1/2 -2 teaspoons chilli flakes (depending on how hot you like things)
* 2 tablespoons cumin seeds
* 2 tablespoons turmeric
* Splash of water
* 2 x 400g tins sliced tomatoes
* 2 tablespoons unsweetened cocoa powder (or cacao)
* If you prefer) consisting of the chickpea water DON'T DRAIN!!
* 2 yellow peppers (or whatever colour you prefer!), 2 x 400g tins chickpeas (or kidney beans,sliced into bitesize pieces
* 2 tablespoons parsley plus additional for garnish Salt and pepper to taste (optional) Side salad (optional)

Prefirst heat the microwave to 400F, meanwhile you can prepare all your things required. When the microwave is hot sufficient location your baking potatoes in the microwave and cook for 1 hour or until they are done how you like them. When the potatoes are in the microwave, position the olive oil and chopped red onion in a big broad pan and cook carefully, with the lid on for 5 minutes, till the onions are not brown however soft. Remove the cover and include the garlic, chilli, ginger and cumin. Cook for a more minute on a low first heat, then consist of the turmeric and a really small splash of water and cook for another minute, taking care not to let the pan get too dry. Next, include in the tomatoes, cocoa powder (or cacao), chickpeas (consisting of the chickpea water) and yellow pepper. Bring to the boil, then simmer on a low very first heat for 45 minutes till the sauce is thick and unctuous (but do not let it burn!). The stew must be done at roughly the same time as the potatoes. Stir in the 2 tablespoons of parsley, and some salt and pepper if you wish, and meal out the stew on top of the baked potatoes, maybe with a basic side salad.

135. Fragrant Asian Hotpot

Preparation time: 10 minutes - Cooking time: 10 minutes
* 1 tea spoon tomato purée
* 1 star anise, crushed (or 1/4 tea spoon ground anise) Small handful (10g) parsley, stalks carefully chopped Little handful (1Og) coriander, stalks finely sliced Juice of 1/2 lime.
* 500ml chicken stock, fresh or made with 1 cube 1/2 carrot, peeled and cut into matchsticks 50g broccoli, cut into little florets 50g beansprouts
* 100 g raw tiger prawns
* 100 g company tofu, sliced

* 50g rice noodles, prepared according to packet actions
* 50g prepared water chestnuts, drained pipes
* 20g sushi ginger, chopped
* 1 table spoon good-quality miso paste

Location the tomato purée, star anise, parsley stalks, coriander stalks, lime juice and chicken
stock in a big pan and bring to a simmer for 10 minutes. Consist of the carrot, broccoli, prawns, tofu, noodles and water chestnuts and simmer gently up until the prawns are cooked through. Get rid of from the first heat and stir in the sushi ginger and miso paste.

Dispense sprinkled with the parsley and coriander leaves.

136. Chargrilled Beef With A Red Wine Jus, Onion Rings, Garlic Kale And Herb Roasted Potatoes

Preparation time: 10 minutes - Cooking time: 50 minutes
* 100g potatoes, peeled and cut into 2cm dice
* 1 table spoon extra virgin olive oil
* 5g parsley, carefully sliced
* 50g red onion, sliced into rings
* 50g kale, sliced
* 1 garlic clove, carefully chopped
* 120-- 150g x 3.5cm-thick beef fillet steak or 2cm-thick sirloin steak
* 40ml red white wine
* 150ml beef stock
* 1 tea spoon tomato purée
* 1 tea spoon cornflour, liquified in 1 table spoon water

First heat the microwave to 440F/ gas 7.
Location the potatoes in a saucepan of boiling water, bring back to the boil and cook for 4-- 5
minutes, then drain. Location in a roasting tin with 1 teaspoon of the oil and roast in the hot
microwave oven for 35-- 45 minutes.
Fry the onion in 1 teaspoon of the oil over a medium first heat for 5-- 7 minutes, until soft and well caramelised. Fry the garlic gently in 1/2 teaspoon of oil for 1 minute, up until soft but not coloured. Include the kale and fry for a further 1-- 2 minutes, till tender. First heat an microwave ovenproof fry pan over a high first heat up until smoking cigarettes.
Cover the meat in 1/2 a teaspoon of the oil and fry in the hot pan over a medium-- high first heat according to how you like your meat done.If you like your meat medium it would be better to sear the meat and then move the pan to a microwave set at 440F/ gas 7 and finish the cooking that method for the prescribed times. Eliminate the meat from the pan and set aside to rest. Consist of the red wine to the hot pan to bring up any meat residue. Bubble to decrease the red wine by half, until syrupy and with a concentrated taste. Consist of the stock and tomato purée to the steak pan and give the boil, then include the cornflour paste to thicken your sauce, including it a little at a time until you have your desired consistency. Stir in any of the juices from the rested steak and dispense with the roasted potatoes, kale, onion rings and red wine sauce.

137. Kale, Edamame, and Tofu Curry

Preparation time: 10 minutes - Cooking time: 50 minutes
* 1 table spoon rapeseed oil
* 1 big onion, chopped

- 4 cloves garlic, peeled and grated
- 1 large thumb (7cm) fresh ginger, peeled and grated
- 1 red chilli, deseeded and thinly sliced
- 1/2 tea spoon ground turmeric
- 1/4 tea spoon cayenne pepper
- 1 tea spoon paprika
- 1/2 tea spoon ground cumin
- 1 tea spoon salt
- 250g dried red lentils
- 1 litre boiling water
- 50g frozen soya edamame beans
- 200g company tofu, chopped into cubes 2 tomatoes, approximately sliced Juice of 1 lime
- 200g kale leaves, stalks eliminated and torn

Include the onion and cook for 5 minutes prior to including the garlic, chilli and ginger and
cooking for a further 2 minutes. Stir through before including the red lentils and stirring once again.
Put in the boiling water and bring to a hearty simmer for 10 minutes, then minimize the very first heat and cook for a further 20-30 minutes till the curry has a thick '- porridge' consistency.
Consist of the soya beans, tofu and tomatoes and cook for a further 5 minutes. Consist of the lime juice and kale leaves and cook until the kale is simply tender.

138. Sirtfood Mushroom Scramble Eggs

Preparation time: 10 minutes - Cooking time: 10 minutes
- 2 eggs.
- 1 tea spoon ground turmeric
- 1 teaspoon mild curry powder
- 20g kale, roughly sliced
- 1 tea spoon additional virgin olive oil
- 1/2 bird's eye chilli, very finely sliced
- handful of button mushrooms, very finely sliced 5g parsley, carefully chopped
- optional Include a seed mixture as a topper and some Rooster Sauce for taste.

Mix the turmeric and curry powder and consist of a little water until you have achieved a light paste.
Steam the kale for 2-- 3 minutes.
Heat the oil in a frying pan over a medium very first heat and fry the chilli and mushrooms for 2-- 3 minutes up until they have actually begun to brown and soften.

139. Fragrant Chicken Breast with Kale, Red Onion, and Salsa-Sirtfood

Preparation time: 10 minutes - Cooking time: 15 minutes
- 120g skinless, boneless chicken breast
- 2 tea spoon ground turmeric
- juice of 1/4 lemon
- 1 table spoon additional virgin olive oil
- 50g kale, chopped.
- 20g red onion, sliced
- 1 tea spoon chopped fresh ginger
- 50g buckwheat

To make the salsa, remove the eye from the tomato and slice it really finely, taking care to keep as much of the l iq uid as possible. Blend with the chilli, capers, parsley and lemon juice. You might put everything in the end however a blender outcome is a bit different. First heat the microwave oven to 440F/ gas 7. Marinate the chicken breast in 1 teaspoon of the turmeric, a little oil and the lemon juice. Leave for 5-- 10 minutes.
Very first heat an microwave ovenproof frying pan until hot, then include the marinated chicken and cook for a minute approximately on each side, up until pale golden, then transfer to the microwave (put on a baking tray if your pan isn't microwave ovenproof) for 8-- 10 minutes or till prepared through. Eliminate from the microwave, cover with foil and leave to rest for 5 minutes before serving.
Prepare the kale in a steamer for 5 minutes. Fry the red onions and the ginger in a little oil, up until soft however not coloured, then consist of the prepared kale and fry for another minute. Cook the buckwheat according to the packet actions with the staying teaspoon of turmeric. Dish outalongside the chicken, vegetables and salsa.

140. Smoked Salmon Omelette

Preparation time: 10 minutes- Cooking time: 10 minutes
- 2 Medium eggs
- 100 g Smoked salmon, sliced
- 1/2 tea spoon Capers
- 10 g Rocket, chopped
- 1 teaspoon Parsley, sliced
- 1 tea spoon Extra virgin olive oil

Split the eggs into a bowl and blend well. Include the salmon, capers, rocket and parsley.
Very first heat the olive oil in a non-stick fry pan up until hot however not cigarette smoking.
Consist of the egg mix and, using a spatula or fish piece, move the mix around the pan until it is even. Reduce the first heat and let the omelette cook through. Slide the spatula around the edges and roll up or fold the omelette in half to dispense.

141. Sirt Food Miso Marinated Cod with Stir-Fried Greens & Sesame

Preparation time: 10 minutes- Cooking time: 15 minutes
- 20g miso
- 1 table spoon mirin
- 1 tablespoon extra virgin olive oil
- 200g skinless cod fillet
- 20g red onion, sliced
- 40g celery, sliced
- 1 garlic clove, finely sliced
- 1 bird's eye chilli, finely sliced
- 1 tea spoon finely chopped fresh ginger
- 60g green beans
- 50g kale, approximately sliced
- 1 tea spoon sesame seeds
- 5g parsley, roughly chopped
- 1 table spoon tamari
- 30g buckwheat
- 1 tea spoon ground turmeric

Mix the miso, mirin and 1 teaspoon of the oil. Rub all over the cod and delegate marinate for 30 minutes. Heat the microwave oven to 440F/ gas 7. Bake the cod for 10 minutes. Include the onion and stir-fry for a few minutes, then consist of the celery, garlic, chilli, ginger, green beans and kale. You might require to consist of a little water to the pan to help the cooking process. Prepare the buckwheat according to the packet steps with the turmeric for 3 minutes. Consist of the sesame seeds, parsley and tamari to the stir-fry and meal outwith the greens and fish.

142. Vietnamese Turmeric Fish with Herbs & Mango Sauce-New

Preparation time: 15 minutes - Cooking time: 30 minutes
Fish:
- 1 1/4 pounds fresh cod boneless, skinless and fish, cut into 2-inch piece large that have to do
- with 1/2 inch thick
- If essential), * 2 table spoon coconut oil to pan-fry the fish (plus a couple of more tablespoon
- Small pinch of sea salt to taste
- Fish marinade: (Marinate for at least 1 hr. or as long as overnight)
- 1 table spoon turmeric powder
- 1 teaspoon sea salt
- 1 table spoon Chinese cooking red wine (Alt. dry sherry)
- 2 tea spoon minced ginger
- 2 table spoon olive oil
- Instilled Scallion and Dill Oil:
- 2 cups scallions (piece into long thin shape)
- 2 cups of fresh dill
- Pinch of sea salt to taste

Mango dipping sauce:
- 1 medium sized ripe mango
- 2 table spoon rice vinegar
- Juice of 1/2 lime
- 1 garlic clove
- 1 tea spoon dry red chili pepper (stir in prior to serving)

Toppings:
- Fresh cilantro (as much as you like)
- Lime juice (as much as you like)
- Nuts (cashew or pine nuts)

1. Marinade the fish for a minimum of 1 hr. or as long as over night.
2. Location all things r eq uired under "Mango Dipping Sauce" into a food mill and blend till wanted consistency.

To Pan-Fry The Fish:
First heat 2 table spoon of coconut oil in a non-stick big frying pan over high very first heat.
When hot, consist of the pre-marinated fish. * Note: place the fish slices into the pan individually and separate to two or more batches to pan fry if essential. You should hear a loud sizzle, after which you can reduce the very first heat to medium-high. Do not move the fish or turn up until you see a golden brown color on the side, about 5 minutes.
Season with a pinch of sea salt. Consist of of more coconut oil to pan-fry the fish is essential.* Note: There need to be some oil left in the frying pan. We utilize the remainder of the oil to make scallion and dill instilled oil.

To Make The Scallion And Dill Infused Oil:.
Utilize the rest of the oil in the fry pan over medium-high first heat, include 2 cups of scallions and 2 cups of dill. Once you have actually includeed the scallions and dill, turn off the first heat.
Provide a gentle toss just up until the scallions and dill have actually wilted, about 15 seconds. Season with a dash of sea salt.
Pour the scallion, dill, and instilled oil over the fish and dish outwith mango dipping sauce with fresh cilantro, lime, and nuts.

143. Moroccan Spiced Eggs

Preparation time: 10 minutes - Cooking time: 15 minutes
- 1 tea spoon olive oil
- 1 shallot, peeled and finely chopped
- 1 red (bell) pepper, deseeded and finely sliced
- 1 garlic clove, peeled and carefully chopped
- 1 courgette (zucchini), peeled and finely chopped
- 1 table spoon tomato puree (paste)
- 1/2 tea spoon mild chilli powder
- 1/4 tea spoon ground cinnamon
- 1/4 tea spoon ground cumin
- 1/2 tea spoon salt
- 1 × 400g (14oz) can sliced tomatoes.
- 1 x 400g (14oz) can chickpeas in water.
- small handful of flat-leaf parsley (10g (1/3oz)), sliced.
- 4 medium eggs at room temperature.

- First heat the oil in a saucepan, include the shallot and red (bell) pepper and fry carefully for 5 minutes. Include the garlic and courgette (zucchini) and cook for another minute or two. Consist of the tomato puree (paste), spices and salt and stir through.
- Include the chopped tomatoes and chickpeas (soaking alcohol and all) and increase the very
first heat to medium. With the cover off the pan, simmer the sauce for 30 minutes-- make sure it is gently bubbling throughout and permit it to minimize in volume by about one-third.
- Remove from the very first heat and stir in the chopped parsley.
- Prefirst heat the microwave oven to 200C/180C fan/350F.
- When you are prepared to cook the eggs, bring the tomato sauce as much as a gentle simmer and transfer to a little microwave oven-proof meal.
- Crack the eggs on the side of the meal and lower them gently into the stew. Cover with foil and bake in the microwave oven for 10-15 minutes. Meal outthe concoction in individual bowls with the eggs drifting on the top.

144. Savory Sirtfood Salmon

- Salmon, 5 oz
- Lemon juice, 1 tbsp
- Ground turmeric, 1 tsp
- Extra virgin olive oil, 2 tbsp
- 1 chopped red onion
- 1 finely chopped garlic clove
- 1 finely chopped bird's eye chili
- Quinoa, 2 oz
- Finely chopped ginger, fresh, 1 tsp
- Celery, chopped, 1 cup
- Parsley, chopped, 1 tbsp
- Tomato, diced, 4.5 oz
- Vegetable stock, 100 ml

Preheat your oven to 200 °C. Fry the celery, chili, garlic, onion, and ginger on olive oil up to three minutes. Add quinoa, tomatoes, and the chicken stock and let simmer for another ten minutes. Layer olive oil, lemon juice, and turmeric on top of the salmon and bake for ten minutes. Add parsley and celery before serving.

145. Sirtfood Miso Salmon

Planning time: 15 min. - Cooking time: 30 min. - Servings: 4
- Miso, 1/2 cup

- Organic red wine, 1 tbsp
- Extra virgin olive oil, 1 tbsp
- Salmon, 7 oz
- 1 sliced red onion
- Celery, sliced, 1 cup
- 2 finely chopped garlic cloves
- 1 finely chopped bird's eye chili
- Ground turmeric, 1 tsp
- Freshly chopped ginger, 1 tsp
- Green beans, 1 cup
- Kale, finely chopped, 1 cup
- Sesame seeds. 1 tsp
- Soy sauce, 1 tbsp
- Buckwheat, 2 tbsp

Marinate the salmon in the mix of red wine, 1 tsp of extra virgin olive oil, and miso for 30 minutes. Preheat the oven to 420 ºF and bake for 10 minutes with the cod.
Fry the onions, chili, garlic, green beans, ginger, kale, and celery for a few minutes until it's cooked. Insert the soy sauce, parsley, and sesame seeds. Cook buckwheat per instructions and mix in with the stir-fry.

146. Sirtfood Salmon with Kale Salad

Planning time: 15 min. - Cooking time: 18 min. - Servings: 4
- Salmon, 4 oz
- 2 sliced red onions
- Parsley, chopped, 1 oz
- Cucumber, 2 oz
- 2 sliced radishes
- Spinach, ½ cup
- Salad leaves, ½ cup

Salad dressing
- Raw honey, 1 tsp
- Greek yogurt, 1 tbsp
- Lemon juice, 1 tbsp
- Chopped mint leaves, 2 tbsp
- A pinch of salt
- A pinch of pepper

Preheat your oven to 200 ºC. Bake the salmon for up to 18 minutes and set aside. Mix in the ingredients for dressing and leave to sit between five and ten minutes.
Serve the salad with spinach and top with parsley, onions, cucumber, and radishes.

147. Spicy Sirtfood Ricotta

- Extra virgin olive oil, 2 tsp
- Unsalted ricotta cheese, 200 g
- Pinch of salt
- Pinch of pepper
- 1 chopped red onion
- 1 tsp of fresh ginger
- 1 finely sliced garlic clove
- 1 finely sliced green chili
- 1 cup diced cherry tomatoes
- ½ tsp ground cumin
- ½ tsp ground coriander
- ½ tsp mild chili powder Chopped parsley, ½ cup Fresh spinach leaves, 2 cup

Heat olive oil in a lidded pan over high heat. Toss in the ricotta cheese, seasoning it with pepper and sea salt. Fry until it turns golden and removes it from the pan. Add the onion to the pan and reduce the heat. Fry the onion with chili, ginger, and garlic for around eight minutes and add the chopped tomatoes. Using the lid to cover and cook for another five minutes.
Add the remaining spices and sea salt to the cheese, put the cheese back into the pan and stir, adding spinach, coriander, and parsley. Use the lid to cover and cook for another two minutes.

148. Vietnamese Turmeric Fish with Herbs & Mango Sauce

Fish:
- Fresh codfish, boneless one ¼ lb
- coconut oil 2 tbsp
- A little pinch of sea salt
- Marinading fish: (Marinate for at least 1 hr. or as long as overnight)
- Turmeric powder 1 tbsp
- Sea salt 1 tsp
- Chinese cooking wine 1 tbsp
- Minced ginger 2 tsp
- Olive oil 2 tbsp
- Infused Scallion and Dill Oil:
- Scallions 2 cups
- Dill 2 cups of fresh
- Pinch of sea salt

Mango dipping sauce:
- Ripe mango one medium-sized
- Rice vinegar 2 tbsp
- Juice of ½ lime
- Garlic one clove
- Dry red chili pepper 1 tsp

1. Marinate the fish for at least 1 hour or overnight for as long as practicable.
2. Put all ingredients in a food processor under "Mango Dipping Sauce" and blend until consistency is desired.
To the Fish Pan-Fry:
1. In a big, non-stick frying pan over high heat, heat 2 tbsp of coconut oil. Then add the pre-marinated fish when heated. * Note: put the fish slices separately in the pan and if appropriate, divide them into two or three batches to pan fry.
2. A noisy sizzle can be detected, during which you should reduce the medium-high heat.
3. Don't switch or move the fish for around 5 minutes before seeing the golden-brown color on foot. Using a touch of sea salt to season. To pan-fry the fish, if appropriate, add more coconut oil.
4. When the fish is golden brown, gently move the fish to the other side to cook. Move it to a wide plate until it's finished.
*Note: The frying pan may have some oil remaining. To render scallion and dill flavored oil, we use the remainder of the oil.
To make the Flavored Oil Scallion and Dill:
1. Using most of the oil over medium-high heat in the frying pan, then apply 2 cups of scallions and 2 cups of dill. Once you have the scallions and dill attached, switching off the heat, offer them a soft toss for around 15 seconds, only before the scallions and dill have wilted. Season with a dash of salt from the sea.
2. Pour over the fish with the scallion, dill, and flavored oil and serve with new cilantro, lime, and nuts with mango dipping sauce.

149. Sirtfood Chicken Breasts

Prep Time: 15 mins - Cook Time: 15 mins

- 120 g skinless, boneless chicken breast Two tsp. ground Tumeric juice of 1/4 lemon One tbsp. extra virgin olive oil
- 50 g kale, chopped
- Twenty g red onion, chopped
- One tsp. fresh ginger
- 50 g buckwheat
- For the Salsa:
- 130 g tomato
- One bird's eye chili, finely chopped
- One tbsp. capers, finely chopped
- Five g parsley, finely chopped juice of 1/4 lemon

To make the salsa, remove the eye
from the tomato and chop it very thinly, taking care to retain as much of the liquid as possible. Chili, capers, parsley, and lemon juice are mixed together. You could put it all in a blender, but the end result is a little different.

Heat the furnace to 2200C/gas 7. Using 1 teaspoon of turmeric, lemon juice, and a little oil to marinate the chicken breast. Leave yourself for 5-10 minutes.

Heat the ovenproof frying pan until hot, then add the marinated chicken and cook until pale golden on each side for about a minute, then transfer to the oven for 8-10 minutes or until cooked through (place on a baking tray if your pan is not ovenproof). Remove from the oven, cover with foil, and leave for 5 minutes to rest before serving.

Meanwhile, cook the kale for 5 minutes in a steamer. In a little oil, fry the red onions and the ginger until soft but not colored, then stir in the cooked kale and fry for another minute.

Cook the buckwheat with the remaining teaspoon of turmeric according to the packet directions. Serve alongside the salsa, tomatoes, and chicken.

150. Sweet-Smelling Chicken Breast, Kale, Red Onion, and Salsa

Planning time: 55 min - Cooking time: 30 min - Servings: 2
- 120g skinless, boneless chicken bosom 2 teaspoons ground turmeric
- 20g red onion, cut
- 1 teaspoon new ginger, sliced 50g buckwheat ¼ lemon
- 1 tablespoon extra-virgin olive oil 50 g kale, cleaved

To set up the salsa, remove the tomato eye and finely cut. Include the chili, parsley, capers, lemon juice, and blend.

Preheat the oven to 220ºC. Pour 1 teaspoon of the turmeric, the lemon juice, and a little oil on the chicken bosom and marinate. Permit to remain for 5–10 minutes.

Place an ovenproof griddle on the warmth and cook the marinated chicken for a moment on each side to accomplish a pale brilliant color. At that point move the container containing the chicken to the oven and permit to remain for 8–10 minutes or until it is finished. Remove from the oven and spread with foil, put in a safe place for 5 minutes before serving.

Put the kale in a liner and cook for 5 minutes. Pour a little oil in a pan and fry the red onions and the ginger to turn out to be delicate yet not shaded. Include the cooked kale and keep on frying for another minute.

Cook the buckwheat adhering to the bundle's guidelines utilizing the rest of the turmeric. Serve close by the chicken, salsa, and vegetables.

151. Butternut pumpkin with buckwheat

Preparation Time: 5 Minutes - Cooking time: 50 Minutes - Servings: 4
- One spoonful of extra virgin olive oil, one red onion, finely chopped
- One tablespoon fresh ginger, finely chopped
- Three cloves of garlic, finely chopped
- Two small chilies, finely chopped
- One tablespoon cumin
- One cinnamon stick
- Two tablespoons turmeric
- 800g chopped canned tomatoes
- 300ml vegetable broth
- 100g dates, seeded and chopped
- one 400g tin of chickpeas, drained
- 500g butter squash, peeled, seeded and cut into pieces
- 200g buckwheat
- 5g coriander, chopped
- 10g parsley, chopped

Preheat the oven to 400 °.

In a frying pan, heat the olive oil and saute the onion, ginger, garlic, and Thai chili. After two minutes, add cumin, cinnamon, and turmeric and cook for another two minutes while stirring.

Add the tomatoes, dates, stock, and chickpeas, stir well and cook over low heat for 45 to 60 minutes. Add some water as required. In the meantime, mix the pumpkin pieces with olive oil. Bake in the oven for about 30 minutes until soft.

Cook the buckwheat according to the Directions and add the remaining turmeric. When everything is cooked, add the pumpkin to the other ingredients in the roaster and serve with the buckwheat. Sprinkle with coriander and parsley.

Calories per serving 248.1 Total Fat .8.7g Saturated fat per serving 2.6g Monounsaturated fat per serving 1.5g Polyunsaturated fat per serving 4.0g Protein per serving 8.5g

152. Roasted Artichoke Hearts

Preparation Time: 5 minutes - Cooking Time: 40 minutes - Servings: 3
- 2 cans artichoke hearts
- 4 garlic cloves, quartered
- 2 tsp extra virgin olive oil
- 1 tsp dried oregano
- salt and pepper, to taste
- 2-3 tbsp lemon juice, to serve

Preheat oven to 375F.

Drain the artichoke hearts and rinse them very thoroughly.

Toss them in garlic, oregano, and olive oil.

Arrange the artichoke hearts in a baking dish and bake for about 45 minutes tossing a few times if desired.

Add salt and pepper to season and serve with lemon juice.

Nutrition: Calories: 35 Fat: 20 g Carbohydrates: 3 g Protein: 1 g Fiber: 1 g

153. Beef Broth

Preparation Time: 5 minutes - Cooking Time: 40 minutes - Servings: 3
- 4-5 pounds beef bones and few veal bones
- 1 pound of stew meat (chuck or flank steak) cut into 2-inch chunks
- Olive oil
- 1-2 medium red onions, peeled and quartered

- 1-2 large carrots, cut into 1-2-inch segments
- 1 celery rib, cut into 1-inch segments
- 2-3 cloves of garlic, unpeeled
- A handful of parsley stems and leaves
- 1-2 bay leaves
- 10 peppercorns

Heat oven to 375F.

Rub olive oil over the stew meat pieces, carrots, and onions.

Put stew meat or beef scraps, stock bones, carrots, and onions in a large roasting pan.

Roast for approximately 45 minutes in the oven, turning everything halfway through the cooking.

Place everything from the oven in a large stockpot.

Pour some boiling water in the oven pan and scrape up all the browned bits and pour all in the stockpot.

Add parsley, celery, garlic, bay leaves, and peppercorns to the pot.

Fill the pot with cold water, over the top of the bones, to 1 inch.

Bring the stockpot to a regular simmer and then reduce the heat to low, so it just barely simmers. Cover the pan loosely and let it simmer for 3-4 hours, low and slow.

Scoop away the fat and any scum that rises to the surface occasionally.

After cooking, remove the bones and vegetables from the pot. Strain the broth.

Let cool to room temperature and then put in the refrigerator.

The fat will solidify once the broth has chilled.

Discard the fat (or reuse it) and pour the broth into a jar and freeze it.

Nutrition: Calories: 65 Fat: 1 g Carbohydrates: 2 g Protein: 3 g Fiber: 0 g

154. *Salmon and Capers*

Preparation Time: 5 minutes - Cooking Time: 40 minutes - Servings: 3

- 75g (3oz) Greek yoghurt
- 4 salmon fillets, skin removed
- 4 tsp Dijon mustard
- 1 tbsp capers, chopped
- 2 tsp fresh parsley
- Zest of 1 lemon

In a bowl, mix the yoghurt, mustard, lemon zest, parsley, and capers.

Thoroughly coat the salmon in the mixture.

Place the salmon under a hot grill (broiler) and cook for 3-4 minutes on each side, or until the fish is cooked.

Serve with mashed potatoes and vegetables or a large green leafy salad.

Nutrition: Calories: 283 Fat: 25 g Carbohydrates: 1 g Protein: 20 g Fiber: 0 g

155. *Pasta Salad*

Preparation Time: 5 minutes - Cooking Time: 40 minutes - Servings: 3

- A plate of mixed greens ingredients
- 1 box (16 ounces) elbow pasta
- 4 cups of water
- 1 tbsp fit salt
- 2 tbsp olive oil
- ½ cup red onion, diced
- 1 cup simmered red peppers, daintily cut ¼ cup dark olives, cut

- ½ pound (8 ounces) crisp mozzarella, diced
- ½ cup slashed basil
- Red wine vinaigrette ingredients
- 1 box (16 ounces) elbow pasta
- 4 cups of water
- 1 tbsp fit salt
- 2 tbsp olive oil
- ½ cup red onion, diced
- 1 cup simmered red peppers, daintily cut
- ¼ cup dark olives, cut
- ½ pound (8 ounces) crisp mozzarella, diced
- ½ cup slashed basil

Amass pressure top, ensuring the weight discharge valve is in the seal position.

Select pressure and set it to high. Set time to 3 minutes.

Select start/stop to start.

Set up the red wine vinaigrette while the pasta is cooking.

In a blending bowl, join all vinaigrette fixings aside from olive oil.

Gradually speed in the olive oil until wholly joined.

Taste and alter seasonings as wanted.

Put in a safe spot.

At the point when weight cooking is finished, enable the strain to discharge for 10 minutes regularly.

Following 10 minutes, snappy discharge remaining weight by moving the weight discharge valve to the vent position.

Cautiously expel top when the unit has completed the process of discharging pressure.

Evacuate the pot and strain the pasta in a colander.

Move to a bowl and hurl with 2 tbsp of olive oil.

Spot bowl in cooler and enable pasta to cool for 20 minutes.

When pasta has cooled, mix in red onion, broiled peppers, dark olives, mozzarella, and basil.

Delicately crease in the red wine vinaigrette.

Serve quickly or cover and refrigerate for serving later.

Nutrition: Calories: 248 Fat: 6 g Carbohydrates: 36 g Protein: 9 g Fiber: 0 g

156. *Sirtfood Caramel Coated Catfish*

Preparation time: 15 minutes - Cooking time: 45 minutes - Serving: 4

- 1/3 cup water
- 2 tbsps. Fish sauce
- 2 shallots, chopped
- 4 cloves garlic, minced
- 1 1/2 tsps. Ground black pepper
- 1/4 tsp. red pepper flakes
- 1/3 cup water
- 1/3 cup white sugar
- 2 lbs. catfish fillets
- 1/2 tsp. white sugar
- 1 tbsp. fresh lime juice
- 1 green onion, thinly sliced
- 1/2 cup chopped cilantro

Combine fish sauce and 1/3 cup of water in a small bowl; mix and put aside.

Combine together shallots, red pepper flakes, black pepper and garlic in another bowl and put aside.

Heat 1/3 cup of sugar and 1/3 cup of water in a big skillet placed over medium heat, stirring from time to time until sugar becomes deep golden brown. Stir in the fish sauce mixture gently and let the mixture boil. Mix and cook the shallot mixture.

Once the shallots have softened, add the catfish to the mixture.

Cook the catfish with cover for about 5 minutes each side until the fish can be easily flake using a fork. Transfer the catfish to a large plate, place a cover, and put aside. Adjust the heat to high and mix in a half tsp. of sugar.

Stir in any sauce that left on the plate and the lime juice.

Let it boil and simmer until the sauce has cooked down.

Drizzle the sauce on top of the catfish and sprinkle with cilantro and green onions.

Nutrition: Calories per serving: 254 Carbohydrates: 4g Protein: 1g Fat: 0.5g Sugar: 3g Sodium: 96mg Fiber: 1g

157. Lentil Tacos

Preparation time: 10 minutes - Cooking time: 12 minutes - Servings: 8

- 2 cups cooked lentils
- ½ cup chopped green bell pepper
- ½ cup chopped white onion
- ½ cup halved grape tomatoes
- 1 teaspoon minced garlic
- ½ teaspoon garlic powder
- 1 teaspoon red chili powder
- ½ teaspoon smoked paprika
- ½ teaspoon ground cumin
- 8 whole-grain tortillas

Take a large skillet pan, place it over medium heat, add oil, and let it heat.

Add onion, bell pepper, and garlic, stir until mixed, and then cook for 5 minutes until vegetables begin to soften.

Add lentils and tomatoes, stir in all the spices and then continue cooking for 5 minutes until hot.

Assemble the tacos and for this, heat the tortillas until warmed and then fill each tortilla with ¼ cup of the cooked lentil mixture.

Serve straight away.

Nutrition: Calories: 315 Fat: 7.8 g Protein: 13 g Carbs: 49.8 g Fiber: 16.2 g

158. Lentil and Quinoa Salad

Preparation time: 5 minutes - Cooking time: 15 minutes - Servings: 4

- 2 medium green apples, cored, chopped
- 3 cups cooked quinoa
- ½ of a medium red onion, peeled, diced
- 3 cups cooked green lentils
- 1 large carrot, shredded
- 1 ½ teaspoon salt
- 1 teaspoon ground black pepper
- 2 tablespoons olive oil ¼ cup balsamic vinegar

Take a large bowl, place all the ingredients in it and then stir until combined.

Let the salad chill in the refrigerator for 1 hour, divide it evenly among six bowls and then serve.

Nutrition: Calories: 199 Fat: 10.7 g Protein: 8 g Carbs: 34.8 g Fiber: 5.9 g

159. Sloppy Joes

Preparation time: 5 minutes - Cooking time: 15 minutes - Servings: 4

- 2 cups cooked lentils
- 2/3 cup diced white onion
- 1 medium sweet potato, peeled, chopped
- 1 medium red bell pepper, cored, diced
- 1 teaspoon minced garlic
- ¾ cup chopped mushrooms
- 1 teaspoon red chili powder
- 1 teaspoon paprika
- 1 teaspoon ground cumin
- 1 tablespoon brown sugar
- 1 tablespoon Worcestershire sauce
- 1 tablespoon olive oil ½ cup vegetable broth 15 ounces tomato sauce

Take a large pan, place it over medium-high heat, add oil, and then let it heat.

Add onion, bell pepper, garlic, mushroom, and sweet potato, stir until mixed, and then cook for 8 minutes or more until potatoes turn tender.

Add lentils, stir in sugar and all the spices, pour in the tomato sauce and then cook for 3 minutes until thoroughly hot.

Pour in the broth, bring the mixture to a simmer, and then remove the pan from heat.

Ladle the sloppy Joes mixture over the bun and then serve.

Nutrition: Calories: 125.3 Fat: 3.6 g Protein: 2.8 g Carbs: 20.1 g Fiber: 3 g

160. Lentil Burgers

Preparation time: 10 minutes - Cooking time: 10 minutes - Servings: 4

- 2 cups cooked green lentils
- 2 tablespoons chopped white onion
- 4 ounces sliced mushrooms
- 1 teaspoon minced garlic
- 2 teaspoons garlic powder
- 2/3 teaspoon salt
- ½ teaspoon ground black pepper
- 1 tablespoon Worcestershire sauce
- 1 tablespoon yellow mustard
- 2 tablespoons olive oil
- 5 hamburger buns

Place the cooked lentils in a blender, pulse until blended, and then tip the mixture into a medium bowl, set aside until required.

Place 1 tablespoon oil in a medium skillet pan, place it over medium heat, and when hot, add onion, mushrooms, and garlic.

Cook for 3 minutes, spoon the mixture to a food processor, add mustard, Worcestershire sauce, and 1 bun, and then pulse until slightly smooth.

Tip the mushroom mixture to lentil, and then stir until combined.

Add salt, black pepper, and garlic powder, stir until mixed, and then shape the mixture into four patties.

Over medium heat, place a skillet pan, add remaining oil and when hot, add patties and then cook for 3 minutes per side until golden brown.

Arrange the patty on a bun and then serve with favorite condiments.

Nutrition: Calories: 184 Fat: 4 g Protein: 11 g Carbs: 28 g Fiber: 9 g

161. Potato Salad

Preparation time: 5 minutes - Cooking time: 25 minutes - Servings: 4

- 2 medium potatoes
- 2 medium tomatoes, diced

- 2 celery, diced
- 1 green onion, chopped

Place a pan with the potatoes, cover with water, and then place the pan over medium-high heat.

Cook the potatoes for 20 minutes, and when done, drain them and let them cool.

Peel the potatoes, cut them into cubes, and then place them into a large bowl.

Add tomatoes, celery, and green onion, season with salt and black pepper, drizzle with oil and then toss until coated.

Divide the salad between three bowls and then serve.

Nutrition: Calories: 268.5 Fat: 15.8 g Protein: 5 g Carbs: 21 g Fiber: 2.5 g

162. Ginger Brown Rice

Preparation time: 5 minutes - Cooking time: 40 minutes - Servings: 3

- 1 cup brown rice, rinsed
- 1-inch grated ginger
- ½ of Serrano pepper, chopped
- 1 green onion, chopped
- 2 cups of water

Take a medium pot, place it over medium-high heat, and then pour in water.

Add rice, green onion, Serrano pepper, and ginger, bring to a boil, switch heat to medium and then simmer for 30 minutes.

Divide rice among three bowls and then serve.

Nutrition: Calories: 125 Fat: 1 g Protein: 3 g Carbs: 26 g Fiber: 0 g

163. Pasta with kale and Black Olive

Preparation time: 10 minutes - Cooking time: 40 minutes - Servings: 3

- 60 g of buckwheat pasta
- 180 gr of pasta
- Six leaves of washed curly kale
- 20 black olives
- Two tablespoons of oil
- ½ chili pepper

Cut the curly kale leaves into strips about 4 cm wide; cook them in salted boiling water for 5 minutes. Also, add the pasta to the pan. While the pasta is cooking, place the oil and olives in a non-stick pan. Drain the pasta and cabbage (keeping some cooking water aside) and add them to the olives. Mix well, adding, if needed, a little cooking water. Add the chili pepper and keep everything well.

Nutrition: Calories per serving 372.7 Total Fat .28.0g Saturated fat per serving 2.7g Monounsaturated fat per serving 10.0g Polyunsaturated fat per serving 2.1g Protein per serving 3.6g

164. Asparagus Soup

Preparation time: 5 minutes - Cooking time: 28 minutes - Servings: 6

- 4 pounds potatoes, peeled, chopped
- 1 bunch of asparagus
- 15 ounces cooked cannellini beans
- 1 small white onion, peeled, diced
- 3 teaspoons minced garlic
- 1 teaspoon grated ginger
- ½ teaspoon salt
- ¼ teaspoon ground black pepper

- 1 lemon, juiced
- 1 tablespoon olive oil
- 8 cups vegetable broth

Place oil in a large pot, place it over medium heat and let it heat until hot.

Add onion into the pot, stir in garlic and ginger and then cook for 5 minutes until onion turns tender.

Add potatoes, asparagus, and beans, pour in the broth, stir until mixed, and then bring the mixture to a boil.

Cook the potatoes for 20 minutes until tender, remove the pot from heat and then puree half of the soup until smooth.

Add salt, black pepper, and lemon juice, stir until mixed, ladle soup into bowls and then serve.

Nutrition: Calories: 123.3 Fat: 4.4 g Protein: 4.7 g Carbs: 16.3 g Fiber: 4.1 g

165. Kale White Bean Pork chops

Preparation Time: 5 minutes - Cooking Time: 45 minutes - Servings: 4-6

- 3 tbsp extra-virgin olive oil
- 3 tbsp chili powder
- 1 tbsp jalapeno hot sauce
- 2 pounds bone-in pork chops
- Salt
- 4 stalks celery, chopped
- 1 large white onion, chopped
- 3 cloves garlic, chopped
- 2 cups chicken broth
- 2 cups diced tomatoes
- 2 cups cooked white beans
- 6 cups packed kale

Preheat the broiler.

Whisk hot sauce, 1 tbsp olive oil and chili powder in a bowl.

Season the pork chops with ½ tsp salt.

Rub chops with the spice mixture on both sides and place them on a rack set over a baking sheet.

Set aside.

Heat 1 tbsp olive oil in a pot over medium heat.

Add the celery, garlic, onion, and the remaining 2 tbsp chili powder.

Cook until onions are translucent, stirring (approx. 8 minutes).

Nutrition: Calories: 140 Fat: 6 g Carbohydrates: 14 g Protein: 7 g Fiber: 3 g

166. Tuna Salad

Preparation Time: 5 minutes - Cooking Time: 40 minutes - Servings: 3

- 100g red chicory
- 150g tuna flakes in brine, drained
- 100g cucumber
- 25g rocket
- 6 kalamata olives, pitted
- 2 hard-boiled eggs, peeled and quartered
- 2 tomatoes, chopped
- 2 tbsp fresh parsley, chopped
- 1 red onion, chopped
- 1 celery stalk
- 1 tbsp capers
- 2 tbsp garlic vinaigrette

Combine all ingredients in a bowl and serve.

Nutrition: Calories: 240 Cal Fat:15 g Carbohydrates: 7 g Protein: 23 g Fiber: 0 g

167. Turkey Curry

Preparation Time: 5 minutes - Cooking Time: 40 minutes - Servings: 3
- 450g (1lb), turkey breasts, chopped
- 100g (3½ oz) fresh rocket (arugula) leaves
- 5 cloves garlic, chopped
- 3 tsp medium curry powder
- 2 tsp turmeric powder
- 2 tbsp fresh coriander (cilantro), finely chopped
- 2 bird's eye chilies, chopped
- 2 red onions, chopped
- 400ml (14fl oz) full-fat coconut milk
- 2 tbsp olive oil

Heat the olive oil in a saucepan, add the chopped red onions and cook them for around 5 minutes or until soft.
Stir in the garlic and the turkey and cook it for 7-8 minutes.
Stir in the turmeric, chilies and curry powder then add the coconut milk and coriander cilantro).
Bring it to the boil, reduce the heat and simmer for around 10 minutes.
Scatter the rocket (arugula) onto plates and spoon the curry on top.
Serve alongside brown rice.
Nutrition: Calories: 400 Fat:6 g Carbohydrates: 3 g Protein: 14 g Fiber: 0 g

168. Tofu and Curry

Preparation Time: 5 minutes - Cooking Time: 36 minutes - Servings: 4
- 8 oz dried lentils (red preferably)
- 1 cup boiling water
- 1 cup frozen edamame (soy) beans
- 7 oz (½ of most packages) firm tofu, chopped into cubes
- 2 tomatoes, chopped
- 1 lime juices
- 5-6 kale leaves, stalks removed and torn
- 1 large onion, chopped
- 4 cloves garlic, peeled and grated
- 1 large chunk of ginger, grated
- ½ red chili pepper, deseeded (use less if too much)
- ½ tsp ground turmeric
- ¼ tsp cayenne pepper
- 1 tsp paprika
- ½ tsp ground cumin 1 tsp salt
- 1 tbsp olive oil

Add the onion, sauté in the oil for few minutes then add the chili, garlic, and ginger for a bit longer until wilted but not burned.
Add the seasonings, then the lentils and stir
Nutrition: Calories: 250 Fat:5 g Carbohydrates: 15 g Protein: 28 g Fiber: 1 g

169. Chicken and Bean Casserole

Preparation Time: 5 minutes - Cooking Time: 40 minutes - Servings: 3
- 400g (14oz) chopped tomatoes
- 400g (14oz) tinned cannellini beans or haricot beans

- 8 chicken thighs, skin removed
- 2 carrots, peeled and finely chopped
- 2 red onions, chopped
- 4 sticks of celery
- 4 large mushrooms
- 2 red peppers (bell peppers), deseeded and chopped
- 1 clove of garlic
- 2 tbsp soy sauce
- 1 tbsp olive oil
- 1.75 liters (3 pints) chicken stock (broth)

Heat the olive oil in a saucepan, put in garlic and onions and cook for 5 minutes.
Add in the chicken and cook for 5 minutes then add the carrots, cannellini beans, celery, red peppers (bell peppers) and mushrooms.
Pour in the stock (broth) soy sauce and tomatoes.
Bring it to the boil, reduce the heat and simmer for 45 minutes.
Serve with rice or new potatoes.
Nutrition: Calories: 324 Fat: 11 g Carbohydrates: 27 g Protein: 28 g Fiber: 7 g

170. Prawn and Coconut Curry

Preparation Time: 5 minutes - Cooking Time: 35 minutes - Servings: 3
- 400g (14oz) tinned chopped tomatoes
- 400g (14oz) large prawns (shrimps), shelled and raw
- 25g (1oz) fresh coriander (cilantro) chopped
- 3 red onions, finely chopped
- 3 cloves of garlic, crushed
- 2 bird's eye chilies
- ½ tsp ground coriander (cilantro)
- ½ tsp turmeric
- 400ml (14fl oz) coconut milk
- 1 tbsp olive oil
- Juice of 1 lime

Place the onions, garlic, tomatoes, chilies, lime juice, turmeric, ground coriander (cilantro), chilies and half of the fresh coriander (cilantro) into a blender and blitz until you have a smooth curry paste.
In a frying pan, heat the olive oil, add the paste and cook for 2 minutes.
Stir in the coconut milk and warm it thoroughly.
Add the prawns (shrimps) to the paste and cook them until they have turned pink and are thoroughly cooked.
Stir in the fresh coriander (cilantro).
Serve with rice.
Nutrition: Calories: 163 Fat: 8 g Carbohydrates: 8 g Protein: 0 g Fiber: 1 g

171. Moroccan Chicken Casserole

Preparation Time: 5 minutes - Cooking Time: 20 minutes - Servings: 3
- 250g (9oz) tinned chickpeas (garbanzo beans) drained
- 4 chicken breasts, cubed
- 4 Medjool dates halved
- 6 dried apricots, halved
- 1 red onion, sliced
- 1 carrot, chopped
- 1 tsp ground cumin
- 1 tsp ground cinnamon

- 1 tsp ground turmeric
- 1 bird's eye chili, chopped
- 600ml (1 pint) chicken stock (broth)
- 25g (1oz) corn flour
- 60ml (2fl oz) water
- 2 tbsp fresh coriander

Place the chicken, chickpeas (garbanzo beans), onion, carrot, chili, cumin, turmeric, cinnamon, and stock (broth) into a large saucepan.

Bring it to the boil, reduce the heat and simmer for 25 minutes.

Add in the dates and apricots and simmer for 10 minutes.

In a cup, mix the corn flour with the water until it becomes a smooth paste.

Pour the mixture into the saucepan and stir until it thickens.

Add in the coriander (cilantro) and mix well.

Nutrition: Calories: 423 Fat: 12 g Carbohydrates: 0 g Protein: 39 g Fiber: 0 g

172. Chili con Carne

Preparation Time: 5 minutes - Cooking Time: 30 minutes - Servings: 3

- 450g (1lb) lean minced beef
- 400g (14oz) chopped tomatoes
- 200g (7oz) red kidney beans
- 2 tbsp tomato purée
- 2 cloves of garlic, crushed
- 2 red onions, chopped
- 2 bird's eye chilies, finely chopped
- 1 red pepper (bell pepper), chopped
- 1 stick of celery, finely chopped
- 1 tbsp cumin
- 1 tbsp turmeric
- 1 tbsp cocoa powder
- 400ml (14 oz) beef stock (broth)
- 175ml (6fl oz) red wine
- 1 tbsp olive oil

In a large saucepan, heat the oil, add the onion and cook for 5 minutes.

Add in the garlic, celery, chili, turmeric, and cumin and cook for 2 minutes before adding then meat then cook for another 5 minutes.

Pour in the stock (broth), red wine, tomatoes, tomato purée, red pepper (bell pepper), kidney beans and cocoa powder.

Nutrition: Calories: 320 Fat: 21 g Carbohydrates: 8 g Protein: 24 g Fiber: 4 g

173. Tofu Thai Curry

Preparation Time: 5 minutes - Cooking Time: 30 minutes - Servings: 3

- 400g (14oz) tofu, diced
- 200g (7oz) sugar snap peas
- 5cm (2-inch) chunk fresh ginger root, peeled and finely chopped 2 red onions, chopped
- 2 cloves of garlic, crushed
- 2 bird's eye chilies
- 2 tbsp tomato puree
- 1 stalk of lemongrass, inner stalks only
- 1 tbsp fresh coriander (cilantro), chopped
- 1 tsp cumin
- 300ml (½ pint) coconut milk
- 200ml (7fl oz) vegetable stock (broth)
- 1 tbsp virgin olive oil

- juice of 1 lime

In a frying pan, heat the oil, add the onion and cook for 4 minutes.

Add in the chilies, cumin, ginger, and garlic and cook for 2 minutes.

Add the tomato puree, lemongrass, sugar-snap peas, lime juice and tofu and cook for 2 minutes.

Pour in the stock (broth), coconut milk and coriander (cilantro) and simmer for 5 minutes.

Serve with brown rice or buckwheat and a handful of rockets (arugula) leaves on the side.

Nutrition: Calories: 412 Fat: 30 g Carbohydrates: 27 g Protein: 14 g Fiber: 5 g

174. Roast Balsamic Vegetables

- 4 tomatoes, chopped
- 2 red onions, chopped
- 3 sweet potatoes, peeled and chopped
- 100g (3½ oz) red chicory (or if unavailable, use yellow)
- 100g (3½ oz) kale, finely chopped
- 300g (11oz) potatoes, peeled and chopped
- 5 stalks of celery, chopped
- 1 bird's eye chili, deseeded and finely chopped
- 2 tbsp fresh parsley, chopped
- 2 tbsp fresh coriander (cilantro) chopped
- 3 tbsp olive oil
- 2 tbsp balsamic vinegar
- 1 tsp mustard
- Sea salt
- Freshly ground black pepper

Place the olive oil, balsamic, mustard, parsley, and coriander (cilantro) into a bowl and mix well.

Toss all the remaining ingredients into the dressing and season with salt and pepper.

Transfer the vegetables to an ovenproof dish and cook in the oven at 200C/400F for 45 minutes.

Nutrition: Calories: 70 Fat:0 g Carbohydrates: 8 g Protein: 2 g Fiber: 2 g

175. Chickpea Salad

Preparation time: 5 minutes - Cooking time: 0 minutes - Servings: 2

- 1 cup cooked chickpeas
- 16 leaves of butter lettuce
- 1 cup chopped zucchini
- ½ spring onion, chopped
- 1 cup chopped celery
- 1 cup grated carrot
- 1 tablespoon chopped cilantro
- ½ teaspoon salt
- ½ tablespoon lemon juice

Take a large bowl, place all the ingredients in it, toss until mixed, and let it sit for 15 minutes.

Divide the lettuce leaves between two portions, top with the salad evenly and then serve.

 Nutrition: Calories: 166.6 Fat: 7.7 g Protein: 4.4 g Carbs: 20.8 g Fiber: 4.3 g

176. Vinaigrette

Preparation Time: 5 minutes - **Cooking Time:** 0 minutes - **Servings:** 1 cup

- 4 teaspoons Mustard yellow

- 4 tablespoon White wine vinegar
- 1 teaspoon Honey
- 165 ml Olive oil

1. In a bowl with a fork, whisk the mustard, vinegar, and honey until well combined.
2. Add the olive oil in small amounts while whisking with a whisk until the vinaigrette is thick.
3. Season with salt and pepper.

Nutrition: Calories: 45 Cal Fat: 0.67 g Carbs: 7.18 g Protein: 0.79 g Fiber: 0.8 g

177. Spicy Ras-El-Hanout Dressing

Preparation Time: 10 minutes - **Cooking Time:** 5 minutes - **Servings:** 1 cup
- 125 ml Olive oil
- 1 piece Lemon (the juice)
- 2 teaspoons Honey
- 1 ½ teaspoons Ras el Hanout
- ½ pieces Red pepper

1. Remove the seeds from the chili pepper.
2. Chop the chili pepper as finely as possible.
3. Place the pepper in a bowl with lemon juice, honey, and Ras-El-Hanout and whisk with a whisk.
4. Then add, drop by drop, the olive oil while continuing to whisk.

Nutrition: Calories: 81 Cal Fat: 0.86 g Carbs: 20.02 g Protein: 1.32 g Fiber: 0.9 g

178. Chicken Rolls With Pesto

Preparation Time: 15 minutes - **Cooking Time:** 20 minutes - **Servings:** 4
- 2 tablespoon Pine nuts
- 25 g Yeast flakes
- 1 clove Garlic (chopped)
- 15 g fresh basil
- 85 ml Olive oil
- 2 pieces Chicken breast

1. Preheat the oven to 175 ° C.
2. Bake the pine nuts in a dry pan over medium heat for 3 minutes until golden brown. Place on a plate and set aside.
3. Put the pine nuts, yeast flakes and garlic in a food processor and grind them finely.
4. Add the basil and oil and mix briefly until you get a pesto.
5. Season with salt and pepper.
6. Place each piece of chicken breast between 2 pieces of cling film
7. Beat with a saucepan or rolling pin until the chicken breast is about 0.6 cm thick.
8. Remove the cling film and spread the pesto on the chicken.
9. Roll up the chicken breasts and use cocktail skewers to hold them together.
10. Season with salt and pepper.
11. In a saucepan, melt the coconut oil and brown the chicken rolls over high heat on all sides.
12. In a baking dish, place the chicken rolls, place in the oven and bake for 15-20 minutes until they are done.
13. Slice the rolls diagonally and serve with the rest of the pesto.

Nutrition: Calories: 105 Cal Fat: 54.19 g Carbs: 6.53 g Protein: 127 g Fiber: 1.9 g

179. Vegetarian Curry From The Crock Pot

Preparation Time: 6 hours 10 minutes - **Cooking Time:** 6 hours - **Servings:** 2
4 pieces Carrot
- 2 pieces Sweet potato
- 1 piece Onion
- 3 cloves Garlic
- 2 tablespoon Curry powder
- 1 teaspoon Ground caraway (ground)
- ¼ teaspoon Chili powder
- 1/4 TL Celtic sea salt
- 1 pinch Cinnamon
- 100 ml Vegetable broth
- 400 g Tomato cubes (can)
- 250 g Sweet peas
- 2 tablespoon Tapioca flour

1. Roughly chop vegetables and potatoes and press garlic. Halve the sugar snap peas.
2. Put the carrots, sweet potatoes and onions in the slow cooker.
3. Mix tapioca flour with curry powder, cumin, chili powder, salt and cinnamon and sprinkle this mixture on the vegetables.
4. Pour the vegetable broth over it.
5. Cover the slow-cooker lid and let it simmer for 6 hours on a low setting.
6. Stir in the tomatoes and sugar snap peas for the last hour.
7. Cauliflower rice is a great addition to this dish.

Nutrition: Calories: 397 kcal Protein: 9.35 g Fat: 6.07 g Carbohydrates: 81.55 g

180. Fried Cauliflower Rice

Preparation Time: 20 minutes - **Cooking Time:** 25 minutes - **Servings:** 4
- 1 piece Cauliflower
- 2 tablespoon Coconut oil
- 1 piece Red onion
- 4 cloves Garlic
- 60 ml Vegetable broth cm fresh ginger
- 1 teaspoon Chili flakes
- ½ pieces Carrot
- ½ pieces Red bell pepper
- ½ pieces Lemon (the juice)
- 2 tablespoon Pumpkin seeds
- 2 tablespoon fresh coriander

1. Cut the cauliflower into small rice grains in a food processor.
2. Finely chop the onion, garlic and ginger, cut the carrot into thin strips, dice the bell pepper and finely chop the herbs.
3. In a pan, melt 1 tablespoon of coconut oil and add half of the onion and garlic to the pan and fry briefly until translucent.
4. Add cauliflower rice and season with salt.
5. Pour in the broth and stir everything until it evaporates and the cauliflower rice is tender.
6. Remove the rice from the pan and set it aside.
7. Melt the rest of the coconut oil in the pan and add the remaining onions, garlic, ginger, carrots and peppers.
8. Fry until the vegetables are tender for a couple of minutes. Season them with a little salt.
9. Add the cauliflower rice again, heat the whole dish and add the lemon juice.
10. Garnish with pumpkin seeds and coriander before serving.

Nutrition: Calories: 261 Cal Fat: 35.61 g Carbs: 34.5 g Protein: 10.27 g Fiber: 8.4 g

181. Fried Chicken And Broccolini

Preparation Time: 10 minutes - **Cooking Time:** 15 minutes - **Servings:** 5
- 2 tablespoon Coconut oil
- 400 g Chicken breast
- Bacon cubes 150 g
- Broccolini 250 g

1. Cut the chicken into cubes.
2. In a pan over medium heat, melt the coconut oil and brown the chicken with the bacon cubes and cook through.
3. Season with chili flakes, salt and pepper.
4. Add broccolini and fry.
5. Stack on a plate and enjoy!
Nutrition: Calories: 198 Cal Fat: 64.2 g Carbs: 0 g Protein: 83.4 g Fiber:0 g

182. Braised Leek With Pine Nuts

Preparation Time: 15 minutes - **Cooking Time:** 15 minutes - **Servings:** 4
- 20 g Ghee
- 2 teaspoon Olive oil
- 2 pieces Leek
- 150 ml Vegetable broth
- fresh parsley
- 1 tablespoon fresh oregano
- 1 tablespoon Pine nuts (roasted)

1. Cut the leek into thin rings and finely chop the herbs. Roast the pine nuts in a dry pan over medium heat.
2. Melt the ghee together with the olive oil in a large pan.
3. Cook the leek until golden brown for 5 minutes, stirring constantly.
4. Add the vegetable broth and cook for another 10 minutes until the leek is tender.
5. Stir in the herbs and sprinkle the pine nuts on the dish just before serving.
Nutrition: Calories: 189 Cal Fat: 9.67 g Carbs: 25.21 g Protein: 2.7 g Fiber: 3.2 g

183. Sweet And Sour Pan With Cashew Nuts

Preparation Time: 15 minutes - **Cooking Time:** 20 minutes - **Servings:** 4
- 2 tablespoon Coconut oil
- 2 pieces Red onion
- 2 pieces yellow bell pepper
- 250 g White cabbage
- 150 g bok choi
- 50 g Mung bean sprouts
- 4 pieces Pineapple slices
- 50 g Cashew nuts

For the sweet and sour sauce:
- 60 ml Apple cider vinegar
- 4 tablespoon Coconut blossom sugar
- 1 ½ tablespoon Tomato paste
- 1 teaspoon Coconut-Aminos
- 2 teaspoon Arrowroot powder
- 75 ml Water

1. Roughly cut the vegetables.
2. Mix the arrow root with five tablespoons of cold water into a paste.

3. Then mix in all the other ingredients for the sauce in a saucepan and add the arrowroot paste for binding.
4. Melt the coconut oil in a pan and fry the onion along with it.
5. Add the bell pepper, cabbage, bok choi and bean sprouts and stir-fry until the vegetables become a little softer.
6. Add the pineapple and cashew nuts and stir a few more times.
7. Pour a little sauce over the wok dish and serve.
Nutrition: Calories: 114 Cal Fat: 55.62 g Carbs: 55.3 g Protein: 30.49 g Fiber: 24.1 g

184. Butter Bean and Miso Dip with Celery Sticks and Oatcakes

Preparation Time: 5 Minutes - **Cooking Time:** 55 Minutes - **Servings:** 4
- 2 x 14-ounce cans (400g each) of butter beans, drained and rinsed Three tablespoons extra virgin olive oil Two tablespoons brown miso paste
- Juice and grated zest of
- 1/2 unwaxed lemon
- Four medium scallions, trimmed and finely chopped One garlic clove, crushed
- 1/4 Thai chili, finely chopped celery sticks, to serve Oatcakes, to serve

1. Simply mash the first seven ingredients together with a potato masher until you have a coarse mixture.
2. Serve with celery sticks and oat-cakes as a dip.
Nutrition: Calories 143. Total fat 3 g. Saturated fat Trace. Trans fat 0 g. Monounsaturated fat 2 g. Cholesterol Trace.

185. Spiced Scrambled Eggs

Preparation Time: 5 Minutes - **Cooking Time:** 15 Minutes - **Servings:** 4
- One teaspoon extra virgin olive oil
- 1/8 cup (20g) red onion, finely chopped 1/2 Thai chili, finely chopped Three medium eggs
- 1/4 cup (50ml) milk
- One teaspoon ground turmeric
- Two tablespoons (5g) parsley, finely chopped

1. In a frying pan, heat the oil and cook the red onions and chili until soft but not browned.
2. Whisk together the eggs, milk, turmeric, and parsley.
3. Add to the hot pan and continue cooking over low to medium heat, continually moving the egg mixture around the pan to scramble it and stop it from sticking/burning.
4. When you have achieved your desired consistency, serve.
Nutrition: Calories 218.2. Total fat 15.3 g. Saturated fat Trace 6.3 g. Trans fat 0 g. Monounsaturated fat 5.5 g. Cholesterol Trace. 386.9 mg

186. Shitake Soup with Tofu

Preparation Time: 5 Minutes - **Cooking Time:** 15 Minutes - **Servings:** 4
- 10g dried Wakame algae (instant)
- 1-liter vegetable stock
- 200g shitake mushrooms, sliced
- 120g miso paste
- 400g natural tofu, cut into cubes
- Two spring onions
- One red chili, chopped

1. Bring the stock to boil, add the mushrooms, and cook for 2 minutes. In the meantime, dissolve the miso paste in a bowl

with some warm stock, put it back into the pot together with the tofu, do not let it boil anymore.

2. Soak the Wakame as needed (on the packet), add the spring onions and Tai Chi, and stir again and serve.

Nutrition: Calories 137.4. Total fat 6.7 g. Saturated fat Trace 1.0 g. Trans fat 0 g. Monounsaturated fat 1.8 g. Cholesterol Trace. 0.0 mg

187. *Chicken Curry with Potatoes And Kale*

Preparation Time: 5 Minutes - **Cooking Time:** 45 Minutes - **Servings:** 4

- 600g chicken breast, cut into pieces Four tablespoons of extra virgin olive oil Three tablespoons turmeric Two red onions, sliced
- Two red chilies, finely chopped
- Three cloves of garlic, finely chopped
- One tablespoon freshly chopped ginger
- One tablespoon curry powder
- One tin of small tomatoes (400ml)
- 500ml chicken broth
- 200ml coconut milk
- Two pieces cardamom
- One cinnamon stick
- 600g potatoes (mainly waxy)
- 10g parsley, chopped
- 175g kale, chopped
- 5g coriander, chopped

1. Marinate the chicken in a teaspoon of olive oil and a tablespoon of turmeric for about 30 minutes. Then fry in a high frying pan at high heat for about 4 minutes. Remove from the pan and set aside.

2. In a pan with chili, garlic, onion, and ginger, heat a tablespoon of oil. Boil everything over medium heat and then add the curry powder and a tablespoon of turmeric and cook, stirring regularly, for another two minutes. Add tomatoes, cook for another two minutes until finally chicken stock, coconut milk, cardamom, and cinnamon stick are added. Cook for about 45 to 60 minutes and add some broth if necessary.

3. In the meantime, preheat the oven to 425 °. Peel and chop the potatoes. Bring water to the boil, add the vegetables with turmeric, and cook for 5 minutes. Then pour off the water and let it evaporate for about 10 minutes. Spread olive oil with the potatoes on a baking tray and bake in the oven for 30 minutes.

4. When the potatoes and curry are almost ready, add the coriander, kale, and chicken and cook for five minutes until the chicken is hot.

5. Add parsley to the potatoes and serve with the chicken curry.

Nutrition: Calories 894 Carbs 162g Fat 22g Protein 25g Fiber 26g Net carbs 136g Sodium 2447mg Cholesterol 0mg

188. *Buckwheat Noodles with Salmon And Rocket*

Preparation Time: 5 Minutes - **Cooking Time:** 45 Minutes - **Servings:** 4

- Two tablespoons of extra virgin olive oil One red onion, finely chopped
- Two cloves of garlic, finely chopped
- Two red chilies, finely chopped
- 150g cherry tomatoes halved

- 100ml white wine
- 300g buckwheat noodles
- 250g smoked salmon
- Two tablespoons of capers
- Juice of half a lemon
- 60g rocket salad
- 10g parsley, chopped

1. In a coated pan, heat 1 teaspoon of the oil, add onions, garlic, and chili at medium temperature and fry briefly. Then add the tomatoes and the white wine to the pan and allow the wine to reduce.

2. Cook the pasta according to the directions.

3. Meanwhile, slice the salmon into strips, and when the pasta is ready, add it to the pan together with the capers, lemon juice, capers rocket, remaining olive oil, and parsley and mix.

Nutrition: Calories 320.1 Carbs. 25.2 Fat 13.0 g Protein 27.0 g

189. *Caprese Skewers*

Preparation Time: 5 minutes - **Cooking Time:** 30 minutes - **Servings:** 2

- 4 oz. cucumber, cut in 8 pieces
- 8 cherry tomatoes
- 8 small balls of mozzarella or 4 oz. mozzarella cut in 8 pieces
- 1 tsp. of extra virgin olive oil
- 8 basil leaves
- 2 tsp. of balsamic vinegar
- salt and pepper to taste

1. Use 2 medium skewers per person or 4 small ones.

2. Alternate the ingredients in the following order: tomato, mozzarella, basil, yellow pepper, cucumber and repeat.

3. Mix together the oil, vinegar, salt, and pepper and pour over the skewers with the dressing.

Nutrition: Calories: 280kcal, Fat: 8g, Carbohydrate: 14.g, Protein: 17g

190. *Baked Salmon with Stir Fried Vegetables*

Preparation Time: 20 minutes - **Cooking Time:** 30 minutes - **Servings:** 2

- Grated zest and juice of 1 lemon
- 1 tsp. sesame oil
- 2 tsp. extra virgin olive oil
- 2 carrots cut into matchsticks
- Bunch of kale, chopped
- 2 tsp. of root ginger, grated
- 8 oz. wild salmon fillets
- Salt and pepper to taste

1. Mix ginger lemon juice and zest together. In an oven proof dish, put the salmon and pour over the mixture of lemon ginger.

2. Cover with foil and leave for 30-60 minutes to marinate.

3. Bake the salmon at 375°F in the oven for 15 minutes.

4. While cooking heat up a wok or frying pan then add sesame oil and olive oil.

5. Attach the vegetables and cook for a few minutes, stirring constantly.

6. Once the salmon are cooked spoon some of the salmon marinade onto the vegetables and cook for a few more minutes.

7. Serve the vegetables onto a plate and top with salmon.

Nutrition: Calories 458kcal, Fat 13.2 g Carbohydrate 15.3 Protein 21.4g

191. *Kale and Mushroom Frittata*

Preparation Time: 15 minutes - **Cooking Time:** 30 minutes - **Servings:** 4

- 8 eggs
- ½ cup unsweetened almond milk
- Salt and ground black pepper, to taste
- 1 tbsp. extra virgin olive oil
- 1 red onion, chopped
- 1 garlic clove, minced
- 1 cup fresh mushrooms, chopped
- 1½ cups fresh kale, chopped

1. Preheat oven to 350°F. In a large bowl, place the eggs, coconut milk, salt, and black pepper, and beat well. Set aside.

2. Heat the oil in a large ovenproof pan over medium heat and sauté the onion and garlic for about 3–4 minutes.

3. Add the kale salt, and black pepper, and cook for about 8–10 minutes.

4. Stir in the mushrooms and cook for about 3–4 minutes. Place the egg mixture on top evenly and cook for about 4 minutes, without stirring.

5. Transfer the pan in the oven and bake for about 12–15 minutes or until desired doneness.

6. Remove from the oven and leave to rest before serving for around 3-5 minutes.

Nutrition: Calories 151, Total Fat 10.2 g, Total Carbs 5.6 g, Protein 10.3 g

192. *Trout with Roasted Vegetables*

Preparation Time: 25 minutes - **Cooking Time:** 20 minutes - **Servings:** 2

- 2 turnips, peeled and chopped
- Extra virgin olive oil
- Dried dill
- 1 lemon, juiced
- 2 carrots cut into sticks
- 2 parsnips, peeled and cut into wedges
- 2 tbsp. Tamari
- 2 trout fillets

1. Put the sliced vegetables into a baking tray. Sprinkle with a dash of tamari and olive oil. Heat the oven to 400°F.

2. After 25 minutes, take the vegetables out of the oven and mix well.

3. Put the fish over it. Sprinkle with the dill and lemon juice. Cover with foil, and go back to the oven.

4. Turn down the oven to 375°F and cook till the fish is cooked through for 20 minutes.

Nutrition: Calories 154.0 Total Fat 2.2 g Carbohydrate 14.5 Protein 23.6

193. *Mince Stuffed Peppers*

Preparation Time: 15 minutes - **Cooking Time:** 60 minutes - **Servings:** 4

- 4 oz. lean mince
- ¼ cup brown rice, cooked
- 2 large yellow
- 2 red bell peppers

- 1 tbsp. parmesan
- 2 tbsp. breadcrumbs
- 3 oz. mozzarella
- 1 egg
- ¼ cup walnuts, chopped
- Salt and pepper, to taste
- 2 cups Arugula
- 2 tsp. extra virgin olive oil
- Few drops Lemon juice
- Cooking spray

1. Preheat oven to 350° F.

2. In a bowl mix mince, parmesan, brown rice, egg and mozzarella. Mix well and set aside.

3. Cut peppers lengthwise, remove the seeds, fill them with the mince mix and put them on a baking tray.

4. Distribute breadcrumbs on top and lightly spray with cooking spray to have a crunchy top without adding calories to the recipe.

5. Cook for 50-60 minutes until peppers are soft. Let cool for a few minutes.

6. Serve stuffed peppers with an arugula salad dressed with olive oil, salt and a few drop of lemon.

Nutrition: Calories 375.1 Fat 8.2g Carbohydrate 24.7g Protein 15.3g

194. *Vanilla Parfait with Berries*

Preparation Time: 5 minutes - **Cooking Time:** 0 minutes - **Servings:** 1

- 4 oz. Greek yogurt
- 1 tsp honey or maple syrup
- 1 cup mixed berries, frozen is perfect
- 1 tbsp. buckwheat granola
- ½ tsp Vanilla extract

1. Mix yoghurt, vanilla extract and honey. Alternate yogurt and berries in a jar and top with granola.

2. Frozen berries are perfect if the parfait is made in advance because they release their juices in the yoghurt.

3. As far as granola, you can use a tablespoon of the one on page 88.

Nutrition: Calories: 318, Fat: 5.4g, Carbohydrate: 22.8g, Protein: 21.9g

195. *Arugula Salad with Turkey and Italian Dressing*

Preparation Time: 5 minutes - **Cooking Time:** 30 minutes - **Servings:** 2

- 8oz. turkey breast
- 1 cup arugula
- 1 cup lettuce
- 2 tsp. Dijon mustard
- 1 tbsp. cumin
- 1/2 cup celery, finely diced
- 2 tsp. oregano
- 1/4 cup scallions, sliced
- 2 tsp. extra virgin olive oil
- Salt and pepper to taste

1. Grill the turkey and shred it. Set aside.

2. Mix lettuce and arugula on a plate. Evenly distribute shredded turkey, celery and scallions.

3. Mix all the dressing ingredients: mustard, olive oil, lemon juice, oregano, salt and pepper in a small bowl and pour over the salad just before serving.

Nutrition: Calories: 165 kcal, Fat: 2.9g, Carbohydrate: 13.6g, Protein:26.1g

196. *Creamy Mushroom Soup with Chicken*

Preparation Time: 10 minutes - **Cooking Time:** 40 minutes - **Servings:** 3

- 2 cups vegetable stock
- 8 oz. mixed mushrooms, sliced
- 1 red onion, finely diced
- 1 carrot, finely diced
- 1 stick celery, finely diced
- 4 oz. chicken breast, cubed
- 1 tbsp. extra virgin olive oil
- 3 leaves sage

1. Put 1 tbsp. oil in a skillet and cook chicken until lightly brown. Set aside.
2. Put the mushrooms in a hot pan with 1 tbsp. oil, celery, carrot, onion and sage and cook for 3 to 5 minutes.
3. Add the stock and let it simmer for another 5 minutes, then using a hand blender, blend the soup until smooth.
4. Add the chicken and cook for another 8 to 10 minutes until creamy.

Nutrition: Calories 302.0 Fat 3.5 g Carbohydrate 16.3 Protein 15 g

197. *Super Easy Scrambled Eggs and Cherry Tomatoes*

Preparation Time: 2 minutes -**Cooking Time:** 2 minutes - **Servings:** 1

- 2 Eggs
- 1 tbsp. Parmesan or other shredded cheese Salt and pepper
- ½ cup cherry tomatoes

1. Put eggs and cheese with a pinch of salt and pepper in a jar. Microwave for 30 seconds, then quickly stir with a spoon.
2. Put back in the microwave for 60 seconds and they are a ready to eat with cherry tomatoes.
3. In case you don't own a microwave, cook the scrambled eggs in a skillet for 2 minutes, stirring continuously until done.

Nutrition: Calories: 278, Fat: 5.4g, Carbohydrate: 12.8g, Protein: 18.9g

198. *Lemon Ginger Shrimp Salad*

Preparation Time: 15 minutes - **Cooking Time:** 5 minutes - **Servings:** 2

- 1 cup chicory leaves
- ½ cup arugula
- ½ cup baby spinach
- 2 tsp. of extra virgin olive oil
- 6 walnuts, chopped
- 1 avocado-peeled, stoned, and sliced
- Juice of ½ lemon
- 8 oz. shrimps
- 1 pinch chili

1. Mix chicory, baby spinach and arugula and put them on a large plate.
2. Heat a skillet on medium high temperature, put 1 tbsp. oil and cook shrimps with garlic, chili, salt and pepper until they are not transparent anymore (5 minutes)
3. Blend avocado with oil, lemon juice with a pinch of salt and pepper and distribute the dressing on top.

4. Chop the walnuts, put them on the plate as last ingredient and serve.

Nutrition: Calories: 353, Fat: 4.8g, Carbohydrate: 28.1g, Protein: 28.3g

199. *Lemon Chicken Skewers with Peppers*

Preparation Time: 5 minutes - **Cooking Time:** 15 minutes - **Servings:** 8

- 8 oz. chicken breast
- 2 cups peppers, chopped
- 1 cup tomatoes, chopped
- 3 tsp. extra virgin olive oil
- 1 garlic clove
- ½ lemon, juiced
- ½ tsp paprika
- ½ tsp turmeric
- 1 handful parsley, chopped
- Salt and pepper

1. Cut the breast in small cubes and let it marinate with oil and spices for 30 minutes.
2. Prepare the skewers and set aside.
3. Heat a pan with oil. When hot add garlic and cook 5 minutes, the remove the clove.
4. Add peppers, tomatoes, salt and pepper and cook on high heat for 5-10 minutes.
5. Heat another pan to high heat, when very hot, put the skewers in and cook 10-12 minutes until golden on every side. Serve the skewers alongside the peppers.

Nutrition: Calories: 315 Fat: 20.9g Protein: 15.8g Carbohydrate: 5.4g

200. *Overnight Oats with Strawberries and Chocolate*

Preparation Time: 5 minutes + 8h- **Cooking Time:** 0 minutes - **Servings:** 2

- 2 oz. rolled oats
- 4 oz. almond milk, unsweetened
- 2 tbsp. plain yoghurt
- 1 cup strawberries
- 1 tsp honey
- 1 square 85% chocolate

1. Mix the oats and the milk in a jar and leave overnight. In the morning top the jar with yoghurt, honey, strawberries and chocolate cut in small pieces.
2. It can be prepared in advance and left in the fridge for up to 3 days.

Nutrition: Calories: 258, Fat: 3.3g, Carbohydrate: 29.8g, Protein: 13.6g

DINNER

201. *Carrot, Buckwheat, Tomato & Arugula Salad in a Jar*

Preparation time: 5 Minutes - **Cooking Time:** 30 Minutes - Servings 2

- 1/2 cup sunflower seeds
- 1/2 cup carrots
- 1/2 cup of shredded cabbage

- 1/2 cup of tomatoes
- 1 cup cooked buckwheat mixed with 1 tbsp. chia seeds
- 1 cup arugula

Dressing:
- 1 tbsp. olive oil
- 1 tbsp. fresh lemon juice and pinch of sea salt

1. Put ingredients in this order: dressing, sunflower seeds, carrots, cabbage, tomatoes, buckwheat and arugula.

202. Honey Mustard Dressing

Preparation time: 10 minutes - Cooking time: 0 minutes - Servings: 2
- 4 tablespoon Olive oil
- 11/2 teaspoon Honey
- 11/2 teaspoon Mustard
- 1 teaspoon Lemon juice
- 1 pinch Salt

Mix olive oil, honey, mustard and lemon juice into an even dressing with a whisk.
Season with salt.

203. Warm tomato salad

Preparation time: 5 Minutes - Cooking Time: 10 Minutes - Servings: 4-5
- 4 tomatoes, sliced
- 1 cup cherry tomatoes, halved
- ½ small red onion, very finely cut
- 2 garlic cloves, crushed
- 1 tbsp dried mint
- 2 tbsp extra virgin olive oil
- 1 tbsp balsamic vinegar

Gently heat oil in a nonstick frying pan over low heat. Cook garlic and tomatoes, stirring occasionally, for 4-5 Minutes or until tomatoes are warm but firm. Remove from heat and place in a plate.
Add in red onion, vinegar and dried mint. To taste and serve, season with salt and pepper.

204. Shredded kale and brussels sprout salad

Preparation time: 10 Minutes - Cooking Time: 20 Minutes - Servings: 4-6
- 18-29 brussels sprouts, shredded
- 1 cup finely shredded kale
- 1/2 cup grated parmesan or pecorino cheese 1 cup walnuts, halved, toasted
- 1/2 cup dried cranberries

For the dressing:
- 6 tbsp extra virgin olive oil
- 2 tbsp apple cinder vinegar
- 1 tbsp dijon mustard
- Salt and pepper, to taste

Shred the brussels sprouts and kale in a food processor or mandolin. Toss them in a bowl, top with toasted walnuts, cranberries and grated cheese.
Whisk in the olive oil in a smaller cup, apple cider vinegar and mustard until smooth. Pour over the salad with the sauce, stir and eat.

205. Quinoa and zucchini ribbon salad

Preparation time: 10 Minutes - Cooking Time: 40 Minutes - Servings: 4
- 1 cup quinoa
- 2 cups water
- 1 zucchini, sliced lengthways into thin ribbons (a mandoline is ideal)
- 3-4 green onions, chopped
- 1 cup cherry tomatoes, halved
- 4 oz feta, crumbled or cut in small cubes
- 2 tbsp extra virgin olive oil
- 3 tbsp lemon juice
- Salt, to taste

Heat oil over medium to high heat in a large saucepan. Add zucchini and and cook, stirring, until zucchini is crisp-tender, about 4 minutes. Set aside in a plate.
Wash the quinoa for 1-2 minutes in a fine mesh strainer under running water, then set aside to drain. Bring water to the boil in a medium saucepan over high heat. Attach the quinoa and put it back to the boil. Cover and cook gently, reducing the heat to a simmer, for 15 minutes. Put aside for 5-6 minutes, sealed.
Toss quinoa with zucchini, green onions, tomatoes, lemon juice and olive oil.
Serve warm or at room temperature, with feta cheese topping.

206. Kale white bean pork soup

Preparation time: 5 Minutes - Cooking Time: 45 Minutes - Servings 4-6
allergies: sf, gf, df, ef, nf
- 3 tbsp. Extra-virgin olive oil
- 3 tbsp. Chili powder
- 1 tbsp. Jalapeno hot sauce
- 2 pounds bone-in pork chops
- Salt
- 4 stalks celery, chopped
- 1 large white onion, chopped
- 3 cloves garlic, chopped
- 2 cups chicken broth
- 2 cups diced tomatoes
- 2 cups cooked white beans
- 6 cups packed kale

Preheat the broiler. Whisk hot sauce, 1 tbsp. Olive oil in a bowl and chili powder. Season the pork chops with 1/2 tsp. Salt. Rub chops with the spice mixture on both sides and place them on a rack set over a baking sheet. Set aside.
Heat 1 tbsp. Olive oil in a pot over medium heat. Add the celery, garlic, onion and the remaining 2 tbsp. Chili powder. Cook until onions are translucent, stirring (approx. 8 minutes).
Add tomatoes and the chicken broth to the pot. Cook and stir occasionally until reduced by about one-third (approx.7 minutes). Add the kale and the beans. Decrease the heat to medium, cover and cook until the kale is soft (approx. 7 minutes). If the mixture looks dry, add up to half a cup of water and season with salt.
In the meantime, broil the pork until browned (approx. 4 to 6 minutes). Flip and broil until cooked through. Serve with the kale and beans.

207. Turkey satay skewers

- 250g (9oz) turkey breast, cubed 25g (1oz) smooth peanut butter 1 clove of garlic, crushed
- ½ small bird's eye chilli (or more if you like it hotter), finely chopped ½ teaspoon ground turmeric
- 200mls (7fl oz) coconut milk 2 teaspoons soy sauce

Servings 2 - 431 calories per serving

Combine the coconut milk, peanut butter, turmeric, soy sauce, garlic and chilli. Add the turkey pieces to the bowl and stir them until they are completely coated. Push the turkey onto metal skewers. Place the satay skewers on a barbeque or under a hot grill (broiler) and Cook on each side for 4-5 minutes, until fully cooked.

208. Salmon & capers

- 75g (3oz) greek yogurt
- 4 salmon fillets, skin removed 4 teaspoons dijon mustard
- 1 tablespoon capers, chopped 2 teaspoons fresh parsley
- Zest of 1 lemon

Servings 4 - 321 calories per serving

Mix the yogurt, mustard, lemon zest, parsley and capers together in a dish. Thoroughly coat the salmon in the mixture. Place the salmon under a hot grill (broiler) and cook for 3-4 minutes on each side, or until the fish is cooked. Serve with mashed potatoes and vegetables or a large green leafy salad.

209. Buckwheat and nut loaf

Preparation Time: 15 minutes - **Cooking Time:** 30 minutes - **Servings:** 4

- 225g/8oz buckwheat
- 2 tbsp. olive oil
- 225g/8oz mushrooms
- 2-3 carrots, finely diced
- 2-3 tbsp. fresh herbs, finely chopped e.g., oregano, marjoram, thyme and parsley
- 225g/8oz nuts e.g., hazelnuts, almonds, walnuts
- 2 eggs, beaten (or 2 tbsp. tahini for vegan version)
- Salt and pepper

1. First of all, put the buckwheat in a pan with 350ml/1.5 cups of water and a pinch of salt. Boil it.
2. Cover and boil with the lid on for about 10-15 minutes, until all the water has been absorbed.
3. Meanwhile, in the olive oil, sauté the mushrooms and carrots until tender.
4. Blitz the nuts until well chopped in the food processor.
5. Stir in the eggs and mix the carrots, cooked buckwheat, herbs and chopped nuts. Combine this with some water while using tahini instead of eggs to create a dense pouring consistency before stirring it into the buckwheat.
6. Season it with pepper and salt.
7. Move to a lined or oiled loaf tin and cook for 30 minutes in the oven on gas mark 5/190C until set and just browned on top.

Nutrition: Calories 163 Carbs 23g Protein 6g Fiber 4g

210. Vegetable broth

Preparation time: 5 Minutes - Cooking Time: 40 Minutes - Servings: 6 cups

- 1 tbsp. Olive oil
- 1 large red onion
- 2 stalks celery, including some leaves
- 2 large carrots
- 1 bunch green onions, chopped
- 8 cloves garlic, minced
- 8 sprigs fresh parsley
- 6 sprigs fresh thyme
- 2 bay leaves
- 1 tsp. Salt
- 2 quarts water

allergies: sf, gf, df, ef, v, nf

Chop veggies into small chunks. Add the onion, scallions, celery, carrots, garlic, parsley, thyme, and bay leaves and heat the oil in a soup pot. For 5 to 7 minutes, cook over high heat, stirring occasionally.

Bring it to a boil, then add salt to it. Lower heat and boil 30 minutes, uncovered. Uh, strain. Other ingredients to consider: stalk of broccoli, root of celery

211. Chicken broth

Preparation time: 5 Minutes - Cooking Time: 50 Minutes - Servings 3

- 4 lbs. Fresh chicken (wings, necks, backs, legs, bones)
- 2 peeled onions or 1 cup chopped leeks
- 2 celery stalks
- 1 carrot
- 8 black peppercorns
- 2 sprigs fresh thyme
- 2 sprigs fresh parsley
- 1 tsp. Salt

allergies: sf, gf, df, ef, nf

Put cold water in a stock pot and add chicken. Bring just to a boil. Skim any foam from the surface. Add other ingredients, return just to a boil, and reduce heat to a slow simmer. Simmer for 2 hours. Let cool and strain until room temperature is warm. Keep the broth cool and use or freeze it within a few days. Defrost and boil prior to use.

212. Artichoke, Chicken and Capers

Preparation time: 10 minutes - Cooking time: 55 minutes - Servings: 2

- 6 boneless, skinless chicken breasts
- 2 cups mushrooms, sliced
- 1 (14 ½ ounce) can diced tomatoes
- 1 (8 or 9 ounce) package frozen artichokes
- 1 cup chicken broth
- ¼ cup dry white wine
- 1 medium yellow onion, diced
- ½ cup Kalamata olives, sliced ¼ cup capers, drained
- 3 tablespoons chia seeds
- 3 teaspoons curry powder
- 1 teaspoon turmeric
- 3/4 teaspoon dried lovage Salt and pepper to taste
- 3 cups hot cooked buckwheat

Rinse chicken & set aside.

In a large bowl, combine mushrooms, tomatoes – with juice, frozen artichoke hearts, chicken broth, white wine, onion, olives and capers.

Stir in chia seeds, curry powder, turmeric, lovage, salt and pepper.

Pour half the mixture into your crockpot, add the chicken, and pour the remainder of the sauce overtop.
Cover and bake for 7 to 8 hours on low or 3 1/2 to 4 hours on high.
Serve with hot cooked buckwheat.

213. *Quinoa and avocado salad*
Preparation time: 10 Minutes - Cooking Time: 20 Minutes - Servings: 4
- 1 cup quinoa
- 2 cups water
- 1 large avocado, pitted and sliced
- ¼ radicchio, finely sliced
- 1 small pink grapefruit, peeled and finely cut
- 1 handful arugula
- 1 cup baby spinach leaves
- 2 tbsp extra virgin olive oil
- 2 tbsp lemon juice
- Salt and black pepper, to taste

Wash quinoa in a fine sieve under running water for 2-3 minutes, or until water runs clear. Set aside to drain, then boil it in two cups of water for 15 minutes.
Fluff with a fork and put to cool aside. Stir avocado, radicchio, arugula and baby spinach into cooled quinoa.
Add grapefruit, lemon juice, and olive oil, season with salt and black pepper and stir to combine well.

214. *Quinoa and carrot salad*
Preparation time: 10 Minutes - Cooking Time: 0 Minutes - Servings: 4
- 1 cup quinoa
- 2 cups water
- 4 carrots, shredded
- 1 apple, peeled and shredded
- 1 garlic clove, chopped
- 3 tbsp lemon juice
- 2 tbsp extra virgin olive oil
- Salt, to taste

In a sieve under running water, rinse the quinoa very well and set aside to drain. Boil two cups of water add in quinoa and simmer for 15 minutes. Fluff with a fork and set aside to cool.
In a deep salad bowl, combine the shredded carrots, apple and lemon juice, garlic and salt. Add in the cooled quinoa, toss to combine and serve.

215. *Quinoa, kale and roasted pumpkin*
Preparation time: 10 Minutes - Cooking Time: 20 Minutes - Servings: 4-5
- 1 cup quinoa
- 2 cups water
- 1.5 lb pumpkin, peeled and seeded, cut into cubes
- 2 cups fresh kale, chopped
- 5 oz crumbled feta cheese
- 1 large onion, finely chopped
- 4-5 tbsp extra virgin olive oil
- 1 tsp finely grated ginger
- ½ tsp cumin
- ½ tsp salt

Preheat oven to 350 f. Line a baking tray and arrange the pumpkin cubes on on it. Drizzle with 2-3 Tablespoons of olive oil and salt. Place in the oven and cook for 20-25 minutes, stirring every 10 minutes. Toss to cover.

Heat the remaining olive oil over a medium-high heat in a large saucepan. Sauté the onion gently for 2-3 minutes or until tender. Connect the spices and cook for 1 minute more, stirring.
Wash quinoa under running water until the water runs clear. Boil two cups of water and add the quinoa to the boil. Reduce heat to low, cover, and simmer for 15 minutes. Incorporate kale and cook until it wilts. Gently combine quinoa and kale mixture with the roasted pumpkin and sautéed onion.

216. *Lamb, Butternut Squash and Date Tagine*
Preparation time: 10 minutes - Cooking time: 25 minutes - Servings: 2
- Two tablespoons olive oil
- One red onion, cut
- 2cm ginger, ground
- Three garlic cloves, ground or squashed
- One teaspoon stew pieces (or to taste)
- Two teaspoons cumin seeds
- One cinnamon stick
- Two teaspoons ground turmeric
- 800g sheep neck filet, cut into 2cm pieces
- ½ teaspoon salt
- 100g Medjool dates, hollowed and hacked
- 400g tin hacked tomatoes, in addition to a large portion of a container of water
- 500g butternut squash, chopped into 1cm 3D shapes
- 400g tin chickpeas, depleted
- Two tablespoons new coriander (in addition to extra for decorate)
- Buckwheat, couscous, flatbreads or rice to serve

Preheat your stove to 140C.
Drizzle around two tablespoons of olive oil into an enormous ovenproof pot or cast iron meal dish. Include the cut onion and cook on a delicate warmth, with the cover on, for around 5 minutes, until the onions are mellowed however not dark-coloured.
Add the ground garlic and ginger, bean stew, cumin, cinnamon and turmeric. Mix well and cook for one increasingly minute with the cover off. Include a sprinkle of water if it gets excessively dry.
Next include the sheep pieces. Mix well to cover the onions and flavours with the beef and afterwards include the salt, hacked dates and tomatoes, in addition to about a large portion of a jar of water (100-200ml).
Bring the tagine to the bubble and afterwards put the cover on and put in your preheated stove for 1 hour and 15 minutes.
Thirty minutes before the finish of the cooking time, include the cleaved butternut squash and depleted chickpeas. Mix everything, set the cover back on and come back to the stove for the last 30 minutes of cooking.
When the tagine is prepared, expel from the stove and mix through the cleaved coriander. Present with buckwheat, couscous, flatbreads or basmati rice.

217. *Prawn Arrabbiata*
Preparation time: 10 minutes - Cooking time: 55 minutes - Servings: 2
- 125-150 g Raw or cooked prawns (Ideally ruler prawns)
- 65 g Buckwheat pasta

- 1 tbsp Extra virgin olive oil

For arrabbiata sauce
- 40 g Red onion, finely slashed
- 1 Garlic clove, finely slashed
- 30 g Celery, finely slashed
- 1 Bird's eye bean stew, finely hacked
- 1 tsp Dried blended herbs
- 1 tsp Extra virgin olive oil
- 2 tbsp White wine (discretionary)
- 400 g Tinned slashed tomatoes
- 1 tbsp Chopped parsley

Fry the onion, garlic, celery and bean stew and dried herbs in the oil over a medium-low warmth for 1–2 minutes. Turn the heat up to medium, include the wine and cook for one moment. Include the tomatoes and leave the sauce to stew over a medium-low warmth for 20–30 minutes, until it has a pleasant creamy consistency. Only include a little water on the off chance that you thought the sauce is getting too thick. While the sauce is cooking, carry a container of water to the bubble and cook the pasta as per the bundle guidelines. At the point when prepared just as you would prefer, channel, hurl with the olive oil and keep in the container until required.

Mix them into the sauce on the off that you are using crude prawns and bake for another 3-4 minutes until it has turned pink and dark,including the parsley and serve. If you are utilizing cooked prawns, include them with the parsley, carry the sauce to the bubble and help.

Add pasta to the sauce, blend altogether yet tenderly and serve.

218. Turmeric Baked Salmon

Preparation time: 10 minutes - Cooking time: 50 minutes - Servings: 2
- 125-150 g Skinned Salmon
- 1 tsp Extra virgin olive oil
- 1 tsp ground turmeric
- 1/4 Juice of a lemon

For the fiery celery
- 1 tsp Extra virgin olive oil
- 40 g Red onion, finely slashed
- 60 g Tinned green lentils
- 1 Garlic clove, finely slashed
- 1 cm fresh ginger, finely slashed
- 1 Bier's eye bean stew, finely slashed
- 150 g Celery, cut into 2cm lengths
- 1 tsp Mild curry powder
- 130 g Tomato, cut into eight wedges
- 100 ml Chicken or vegetable stock
- 1 tbsp Chopped parsley

Heat the grill to 200C/gas mark 6.

Start with the fiery celery. Warmth a skillet over medium-low heat, include the olive oil, at that point the onion, garlic, ginger, bean stew and celery. Fry tenderly for 2–3 minutes or until mollified however not hued, at that point include the curry powder and cook for a further moment.

Add the red tomato then the stock and lentils and stew delicately for 10 minutes. You might need to increment or decrease the cooking time contingent upon how crunchy you like your celery.

Meanwhile, blend the turmeric, oil and lemon squeeze and rub over the salmon.

Place on a heating plate and cook for 8–10 minutes.

To complete, mix the parsley through the celery and present with the salmon.

219. Buckwheat with Mushrooms and Green Onions

Preparation time: 10 minutes - Cooking time: 40 minutes - Servings: 2
- 1 cup buckwheat groats
- 2 cups vegetable or chicken broth
- 3 green onions, thinly sliced
- 1 cup mushrooms, sliced
- Salt and pepper to taste
- 2 teaspoons butter

Combine all ingredients in your crockpot. Cover and cook on low for 4 to 4 1/2 hours.

220. Pasta with Cheesy Meat Sauce

Preparation Time: 10 minutes - Cooking Time: 30 minutes - Servings: 6
- ½ box large-shaped pasta
- 1-pound ground beef*
- ½ cup onions, diced
- 1 tablespoon onion flakes
- 1½ cups beef stock, reduced or no sodium
- 1 tablespoon Better Than Bouillon® beef, no salt added
- 1 tablespoon tomato sauce, no salt added
- ¾ cup Monterey or pepper jack cheese, shredded
- 8 ounces cream cheese, softened
- ½ teaspoon Italian seasoning
- ½ teaspoon ground black pepper
- 2 tablespoons French's® Worcestershire sauce, reduced sodium

1. Cook pasta noodles as per the directions on the box.
2. Cook the ground beef, onions and onion flakes in a large skillet until the meat is browned.
3. Add stock, bouillon and tomato sauce and drain.
4. Bring to a boil, sometimes stirring. Stir in the pasta that has been cooked, turn off the heat and add the cream cheese, shredded cheese and flavoured cheese (Italian seasoning, black pepper and Worcestershire sauce). Stir in the pasta mixture until all the cheese is melted.

TIP: You can substitute beef for ground turkey.

Nutrition: Calories: 502 kcal Total Fat: 30 g Saturated Fat: 14 g Cholesterol: 99 mg Sodium: 401 mg Total Carbs: 35 g Fiber: 1.7 g Sugar: 0 g Protein: 23 g

221. Kale, Apple, & Cranberry Salad

Preparation time: 15 minutes - Cooking time: 5 minutes - Servings: 4
- 6 cups fresh baby kale
- 3 large apples, cored and sliced
- ¼ cup unsweetened dried cranberries
- ¼ cup almonds, sliced
- tablespoons extra-virgin olive oil
- 1 tablespoon raw honey
- Salt and ground black pepper, to taste

1. Place all the ingredients in a salad bowl and toss to coat them well.
2. Serve immediately.

222. *Arugula, Strawberry, & Orange Salad*

Preparation time: **15 minutes** - Servings: 4
Salad
- 6 cups fresh baby arugula
- 1½ cups fresh strawberries, hulled and sliced 2 oranges, peeled and segmented

Dressing
- 2 tablespoons fresh lemon juice
- 1 tablespoon raw honey
- 2 teaspoons extra-virgin olive oil
- 1 teaspoon Dijon mustard
- Salt and ground black pepper, to taste

For salad: in a salad bowl, place all ingredients and mix.
For dressing: place all ingredients in another bowl and beat until well combined.
Place dressing on top of salad and toss to coat well.

223. *Minty Tomatoes and Corn*

Preparation time: 10 minutes - Cooking time: 65 minutes - Servings: 2
- 2 c. corn
- 1 tbsp. rosemary vinegar
- 2 tbsps. chopped mint
- 1 lb. sliced tomatoes
- ¼ tsp. black pepper
- 2 tbsps. olive oil

In a salad bowl, combine the tomatoes with the corn and the other ingredients, toss and serve.

224. *Beef & Kale Salad*

Preparation time: **15 minutes** - Cooking time: **8 minutes** - Servings: 2
Steak
- 2 teaspoons olive oil
- 2 (4-ounce) strip steaks
- Salt and ground black pepper, to taste

Salad
- ¼ cup carrot, peeled and shredded
- ¼ cup cucumber, peeled, seeded, and sliced
- ¼ cup radish, sliced
- ¼ cup cherry tomatoes, halved
- 3 cups fresh kale, tough ribs removed and chopped

Dressing
- 1 tablespoon extra-virgin olive oil
- 1 tablespoon fresh lemon juice
- Salt and ground black pepper, to taste

1. For steak: in a large heavy-bottomed wok, heat the oil over high heat and cook the steaks with salt and black pepper for about 3–4 minutes per side.
2. Transfer the steaks onto a cutting board for about 5 minutes before slicing.
3. For salad: place all ingredients in a salad bowl and mix.
4. For dressing: place all ingredients in another bowl and beat until well combined.
5. Cut the steaks into desired sized slices against the grain.
6. Place the salad onto each serving plate.
7. Top each plate with steak slices.
8. Drizzle with dressing and serve.

225. *Salmon Burgers*

Preparation time: **20 minutes** - Cooking time: **15 minutes** - Servings: 5
Burgers
- 1 teaspoon olive oil
- 1 cup fresh kale, tough ribs removed and chopped 1/3 cup shallots, chopped finely
- Salt and ground black pepper, to taste
- 16 ounces skinless salmon fillets
- ¾ cup cooked quinoa
- 2 tablespoons Dijon mustard
- 1 large egg, beaten

Salad
- 2½ tablespoons olive oil
- 2½ tablespoons red wine vinegar
- Salt and ground black pepper, to taste
- 8 cups fresh baby arugula
- 2 cups cherry tomatoes, halved

1. For burgers: in a large non-stick wok, heat the oil over medium heat and sauté the kale, shallots, salt, and black pepper for about 4–5 minutes.
2. Remove from heat and transfer the kale mixture into a large bowl.
3. Set aside to cool slightly.
4. With a knife, chop 4 ounces of salmon and transfer into the bowl of kale mixture.
5. In a food processor, add the remaining salmon and pulse until finely chopped.
6. Transfer the finely chopped salmon into the bowl of kale mixture.
7. Then, add remaining ingredients and stir until fully combined.
8. Make 5 equal-sized patties from the mixture.
9. Heat a lightly greased large non-stick wok over medium heat and cook the patties for about 4–5 minutes per side.
10. For dressing: in a glass bowl, add the oil, vinegar, shallots, salt, and black pepper, and beat until well combined.
11. To coat well, add the arugula and tomatoes and toss.
12. Divide the salad onto on serving plates and top each with 1 patty.

226. *Sirtfood bites*

- 4 oz walnuts
- 1 oz dark chocolate (85 per cent cocoa solids), broken into pieces; or cocoa nibs
- 9 oz Medjool dates, pitted 1 tbsp cocoa powder
- 1 tbsp ground turmeric
- 1 tbsp extra virgin vegetable oil the scraped seeds of 1 vanilla pod or 1 tsp vanilla 1–2 tbsp water

Place the walnuts and chocolate during a kitchen appliance and process until you have a fine powder. Add all the opposite ingredients except the water and blend until the mixture forms a ball. Depending on the consistency of the mixture, you may or may not have to add water-you don't want it to be too wet. Shape the mixture into bite-sized balls using your hands and refrigerate for at least 1 hour in an airtight container before eating them. You'll roll some of the balls in some more cocoa or desiccated coconut to realize a different finish if you wish. They will keep for up to 1 week in your fridge.

227. Asian king prawn stir-fry with buckwheat noodles

- 5 oz shelled raw king prawns, deveined
- 2 tsp tamari (you can use soy sauce if you're not avoiding gluten) 2 tsp extra virgin olive oil
- 2.5 oz soba (buckwheat noodles) 1 clove , finely chopped
- 1 bird's eye chilli, finely chopped 1 tsp finely chopped fresh ginger ¼ red onions, sliced
- 1.5 oz celery, trimmed and sliced 3 oz green beans, chopped
- 2 oz kale, roughly chopped
- ½ cup chicken broth
- 1 tbsp lovage or celery leaves

Over a high heat, heat a frypan, then cook the prawns for 2-3 minutes in 1 teaspoon tamari and 1 teaspoon oil. Transfer the prawns to a plate. Wipe the pan out with kitchen paper, as you're getting to use it again. Cook the noodles in boiling water for 5–8 minutes or as directed on the packet. Drain and set aside.

Meanwhile, fry the garlic, chilli and ginger, red onion, celery, beans and kale within the remaining oil over an medium–high heat for 2–3 minutes. Add the stock and convey to the boil, then simmer for a minute or two, until the vegetables are cooked but still crunchy.

Add the prawns, noodles and lovage/celery leaves to the pan, bring back to the boil then remove from the heat and serve.

228. Strawberry buckwheat tabouleh

- 2 oz buckwheat
- 1 tbsp ground turmeric
- ½ avocado
- ½ tomato
- ¼ red onion
- 1 oz Medjool dates, pitted
- 1 tbsp capers
- 1 oz parsley
- 3 oz strawberries, hulled
- 1 tbsp extra virgin olive oil
- juce of ½ lemon
- 1 oz rocket

Cook the buckwheat with the turmeric consistent with the packet instructions.
Drain and keep to one side to chill.
Finely chop the avocado, tomato, red onion, dates, capers and parsley and blend with the cool buckwheat. Slice the strawberries and gently mix into the salad with the oil and juice. Serve on a bed of rocket.

229. Chicken Skewers with Satay Sauce

- 5 oz pigeon breast, dig chunks 1 tsp. Ground turmeric 1/2 tsp. extra virgin vegetable oil
- 1.5 oz Buckwheat
- 1 oz Kale, stalks removed and sliced 1 oz Celery, sliced
- 4 Walnut halves, chopped, to garnish
- ¼ purple onion , diced 1 clove , chopped
- 1 tsp. Extra virgin vegetable oil 1 tsp. favorer
- 1 tsp. Ground turmeric
- ¼ cup chicken broth ½ cup Coconut milk
- 1 tbsp. Walnut butter or spread 1 tbsp. Coriander, chopped

Mix the chicken with the turmeric and vegetable oil and put aside to marinate 30 minutes to 1 hour would be best, but if you're short on time, just leave it for as long as you'll
Cook the buckwheat consistent with the packet instruc tions, for the last 5-7 minutes of cooking time, the kale and celery are added. Drain. Heat the grill on a high setting.
For the sauce, gently fry the purple onion and garlic within the vegetable oil for 2–3 minutes until soft. Add the spices and cook for an extra minute. Add the stock and coconut milk and convey to the boil, then add the walnut butter and stir through. Reduce the warmth and simmer the sauce for 8 or 10 minutes, or till creamy and rich. As the sauce is simmering, thread the chicken on to the skewers and place under the recent grill for 10 minutes, turning them after 5 minutes. To serve, stir the coriander through the sauce and pour it over the skewers, then scatter over the chopped walnuts.

230. Smoked salmon omelette

- 2 Medium eggs
- 4 oz Smoked salmon, sliced 1/2 tsp. Capers
- 0.5 oz Rocket, chopped 1 tsp. Parsley, chopped
- 1 tsp. Extra virgin olive oil

Crack the eggs into a bowl and whisk well. Add the salmon, capers, rocket and parsley.
Heat the olive oil during a non-stick frypan until hot but not smoking. Add the egg mixture and, employing a spatula or turner, move the mixture round the pan until it's even. Reduce the warmth and let the omelette cook through. Slide the spatula around the edges and roll up or fold the omelette in half to serve.

231. The Sirtfood Diet's Shakshuka

- 1 tsp. extra virgin vegetable oil
- ½ purple onion, finely chopped 1 Garlic clove, finely chopped 1 oz Celery, finely chopped
- 1 Bird's eye chilli, finely chopped 1 tsp. Groud cumin 1 tsp. Ground turmeric 1 tsp. Paprika
- 3 Tinned chopped tomatoes
- 1 oz Kale, stems removed and roughly chopped 1 tbsp. Chopped parsley 2 Medium eggs D

Heat alittle , deep-sided frypan over a medium–low heat.
Add the oil and fry the onion, garlic, celery, chilli and spices for 1–2 minutes.
Add the tomatoes, then leave the sauce to simmer gently for 20 minutes, stirring occasionally.
Add the kale and cook for an extra 5 minutes. If you are feeling the sauce is getting too thick, simply add a touch water. When your sauce features a nice rich consistency, stir within the parsley.
Make two little wells within the sauce and crack each egg into them. Reduce the heat to its lowest setting and canopy the pan with a lid or foil. Leave the eggs to cook for 10–12 minutes, at which point the whites should be firm while the yolks are still runny. Cook for a further 3–4 minutes if you favor the yolks to be firm. Serve immediately – ideally straight from the pan.

232. Chicken with Broccoli & Mushrooms

Preparation time: **15 minutes** - **Cooking** time: **25 minutes** - Servings: 6

- 3 tablespoons olive oil
- 1 pound skinless, boneless chicken breast, cubed

- 1 medium onion, chopped
- 6 garlic cloves, minced
- 2 cups fresh mushrooms, sliced
- 16 ounces small broccoli florets
- ¼ cup water
- Salt and ground black pepper, to taste

1. Over medium heat, heat the oil in a large wok and cook the chicken cubes for around 4-5 minutes.
2. With a slotted spoon, transfer the chicken cubes onto a plate.
3. In the same wok, add the onion and sauté for about 4–5 minutes.
4. Add the fungus and cook for approximately 4-5 minutes.
5. Stir in the cooked chicken, broccoli, and water, and cook (covered) for about 8–10 minutes, stirring occasionally.
6. Stir in salt and black pepper and remove from heat.
7. Serve hot.

233. Buckwheat noodles with chicken kale & miso dressing

For the noodles:
- 2-3 handfuls of kale leaves
- 5 oz buckwheat noodles (100% buckwheat, no wheat) 3-4 shiitake mushrooms, sliced
- 1 tsp copra oil or ghee
- 1 brown onion, finely diced
- 1 medium free-range pigeon breast , sliced or diced 1 long red chilli, thinly sliced
- 2 large garlic cloves, finely diced2-3 tbsp Tamari sauce (gluten-free soy sauce)

For the miso
- dressing: 1½ tablespoon fresh organic miso 1 tbsp Tamari sauce
- 1 tbsp extra-virgin vegetable oil 1 tbsp lemon or juice
- 1 tsp sesame oil (optional)

Bring an medium saucepan of water to boil. Add the kale and cook for 1 minute, until slightly wilted. Remove and set aside but reserve the water and convey it back to the boil. Add the soba noodles and cook consistent with the package instructions (usually about 5 minutes). Rinse under cold water and put aside.

Within the meantime, pan fry the shiitake mushrooms during a little ghee or coconut oil (about a teaspoon) for 2-3 minutes, until lightly browned on all sides. Sprinkle with sea salt and put aside.

Within the same frypan , heat more copra oil or ghee over medium-high heat. Sauté onion and chilli for 2-3 minutes and then add the chicken pieces. Cook 5 minutes over medium heat, stirring a couple of times, then add the garlic, tamari sauce and a touch splash of water. Cook for a further 2-3 minutes, stirring frequently until chicken is cooked through.

Finally, add the kale and soba noodles and toss through the chicken to warm up.

Mix the miso dressing and drizzle over the noodles right at the end of cooking, this manner you'll keep all those beneficial probiotics in the miso alive and active.

234. Baked salmon salad (creamy mint dressing)

- 1 salmon fillet (4 oz)
- 1.5 oz mixed salad leaves
- 1.5 oz young spinach leaves
- 2 radishes, trimmed and thinly sliced 2 oz cucumber, dig chunks
- 2 spring onions, trimmed and sliced
- 1 small handful parsley, roughly chopped

For the dressing:
- 1 tsp low-fat mayonnaise 1 tbsp natural yogurt
- 1 tbsp rice vinegar
- 2 leaves mint, finely chopped
- Salt and freshly ground black pepper

Preheat the oven to 390 °F.

Place the salmon fillet on a baking tray and bake for 16–18 minutes until just cooked through. Remove from the oven and set aside. The salmon is equally nice hot or cold in the salad. If your salmon has skin, simply cook skin side down and remove the salmon from the skin employing a turner after cooking. It should slide off easily when cooked.

During a small bowl, mix together the mayonnaise, yogurt, rice wine vinegar, mint leaves and salt and pepper together and leave to face for a minimum of 5 minutes to permit the flavors to develop.

Arrange the salad leaves and spinach on a serving plate and top with the radishes, cucumber, spring onions and parsley. Flake the cooked salmon onto the salad and drizzle the dressing over.

235. Choco chip granola

- 7 oz jumbo oats
- 2 oz pecans, roughly chopped 3 tbsp light vegetable oil
- 1 oz butter
- 1 tbsp dark sugar
- 2 tbsp rice malt syrup
- 2 oz good-quality (70%) bittersweet chocolate chips

Preheat the oven to 320 °F. Line an outsized baking tray with a silicone sheet or baking parchment.

Mix the oats and pecans together during a large bowl. During a small nonstick pan, gently heat the olive oil, butter, sugar and rice malt syrup until the butter has melted and therefore the sugar and syrup have dissolved. Don't allow to boil. Pour the syrup over the oats and stir thoroughly until the oats are fully covered.

Distribute the granola over the baking tray, spreading right into the corners. Leave clumps of mixture with spacing instead of an even spread. Bake within the oven for 20 minutes until just tinged golden brown at the edges. Remove from the oven and leave to chill on the tray completely.

When cool, hack any bigger lumps on the tray together with your fingers and then mix within the chocolate chips. Scoop or pour the granola into an airtight tub or jar. The granola will keep for a minimum of 2 weeks.

236. Chargrilled beef

- 1 potato, peeled, and dig small dice 1 tbsp extra virgin olive oil
- 1 tbsp parsley, finely chopped
- ½ red onion, sliced into rings 2 oz kale, sliced
- 1 clove, finely chopped
- 4 oz 1½"-thick beef fillet steak or 1"-thick beefsteak 3 tbsp red wine
- ½ cup beef broth 1 tsp tomato purée
- 1 tsp cornflour, dissolved in 1 tbsp water

Heat the oven to 430 °F.

Place the potatoes during a saucepan of boiling water, bring back to the boil and cook for 4–5 minutes, then drain. Place during a roasting tin with 1 teaspoon of the oil and roast in the hot oven for 35–45 minutes. Turn the potatoes every 10 minutes to make sure even cooking. When cooked, remove from the oven, sprinkle with the chopped parsley and mix well.

Fry the onion in 1 teaspoon of the oil over medium heat for 5–7 minutes, until soft and nicely caramelized. Keep warm. Steam the kale for 2–3 minutes then drain. Fry the garlic gently in ½ teaspoon of oil for 1 minute, till soft but not colored. Add the kale and fry for a further 1–2 minutes, until tender. Keep warm.

Heat an ovenproof frypan over high heat until smoking. Coat the meat in ½ a teaspoon of the oil and fry within the hot pan over an medium–high heat consistent with how you wish your meat done.If you like your meat medium, it might be better to sear the meat then transfer the pan to an oven set at 430°F and finish the cooking that the way for the prescribed times.

Remove the meat from the pan and set aside to rest. Add the wine to the hot pan to mention any meat residue — Bubble to scale back the wine by half, until syrupy and with a concentrated flavor. Add the stock and tomato purée to the steak pan and convey to the boil, then add the cornflour paste to thicken your sauce, adding it a little at a time until you've got your desired consistency. Stir in any of the juices from the rested steak and serve with the roasted potatoes, kale, onion rings and wine sauce.

237. Greek Sea Bass Mix

Preparation time: 10 minutes - Cooking time: 22 minutes - Servings: 2

- 2 sea bass fillets, boneless
- 1 garlic clove, minced
- 5 cherry tomatoes, halved
- 1 tablespoon chopped parsley
- 2 shallots, chopped
- Juice of ½ lemon
- 1 tablespoon olive oil
- 8 ounces baby spinach
- Cooking spray

1. Grease a baking dish with cooking oil then add the fish, tomatoes, parsley and garlic. Drizzle the lemon juice over the fish, cover the dish and place it in the oven at 350 degrees F. Bake for 15 minutes and then divide between plates. Heat a pan over medium heat with the olive oil, add shallot, stir and cook for 1 minute. Add spinach, stir, cook for 5 minutes more, add to the plate with the fish and serve.

238. Veal Cabbage Rolls – Smarter with Capers, Garlic and Caraway Seeds

- 1 kg white cabbage (1 white cabbage)
- Salt
- 2 onions
- 1 clove of garlic
- 3 tbsp oil
- 700 g veal mince (request from the butcher)
- 40 g escapades (glass; depleted weight)
- 2 eggs Pepper
- 1 tsp favorer
- 1 tbsp paprika powder (sweet)
- 400 ml veal stock

- 125 ml soy cream

Wash the cabbage and evacuate the external leaves. Cut out the tail during a wedge. Spot a huge pot of salted water and heat it to the aim of boiling. Within the interim, expel 16 leaves from the cabbage during a gentle progression, increase the bubbling water and cook for 3-4 minutes

Lift out, flush under running virus water and channel. Spot on a kitchen towel, spread with a subsequent towel and pat dry Cut out the hard, center leaf ribs.

Peel and finely cleave onions and garlic. Warmth 1 tablespoon of oil. Braise the onions and garlic until translucent.

Let cool during a bowl. Include minced meat, tricks, eggs, salt, and pepper and blend everything into a meat player. Put 2 cabbage leaves together and put 1 serving of mince on each leaf. Move up firmly and fasten it with kitchen string.

Heat the rest of the oil during a pan and earthy colored the 8 cabbage abounds in it from all sides.

Add the caraway and paprika powder. Empty veal stock into the pot and heat to the aim of boiling. Cover and braise the cabbage turns over medium warmth for 35–40 minutes, turn within the center. Mix the soy cream into the sauce and let it bubble for an extra 5 minutes. Season with salt and pepper. Put the cabbage roulades on a plate and present with earthy colored rice or pureed potatoes.

239. Prawns Sweet and Spicy Glaze with China-Cole-Slav

- 250 g Chinese cabbage (0.25 Chinese cabbage)
- Salt
- 50 g little carrots (1 little carrot)
- 1 little red onion
- ½ lime
- 75 ml coconut milk (9% fat)
- 2 tsp sugar
- 1 tsp vinegar
- Pepper
- 2 stems coriander
- 3 tbsp pure sweetener
- 1 dried stew pepper
- 2 tbsp Thai fish sauce
- 1 clove of garlic
- 3 spring onions
- 400 g shrimps (with shell, 8 shrimps)
- 2 tbsp oil

Clean the cabbage and evacuate the tail. Cut the cabbage into fine strips over the rib. Sprinkle with somewhat salt, blend vivaciously and let steep for half-hour.

Within the interim, strip the carrot, dig fine strips. Strip the red onion and furthermore dig strips. Crush the lime.

Mix coconut milk with sugar, vinegar, 1 tbsp juice, and slightly pepper. Channel the cabbage and blend it in with the carrot and onion strips with the coconut milk.

Wash the coriander leaves, shake dry, pluck the leaves, cleave and blend within the plate of mixed greens. Let it steep for an extra half-hour.

Boil the natural sweetener, stew pepper, fish sauce, and three tablespoons of water during a touch pot and cook while mixing until the sugar has totally weakened. Allow chill to off.

Peel and smash garlic. The spring onions are washed and cleaned and cut into pieces about 2 cm long.

Break the shrimp out of the shells, however, leave the rear ends on the shrimp.

Cut open the rear, evacuate the dark digestion tracts. Wash shrimp and pat dry.

Heat oil within the wok and to the aim of smoke. Include the shrimp and garlic and fry quickly. Season with pepper.

Add 3-4 tablespoons of the bean stew fish sauce and cook while mixing until the sauce adheres to the shrimp; that takes around 2 minutes.

Add the onion pieces and fry for an extra 45 seconds. Season the coleslaw once more. Put the shrimp on a plate and present it with the serving of mixed greens.

240. Vegetarian Lasagna - Smarter with Seitan and Spinach

- 225 g spinach leaves (solidified)
- 300 g seitan
- 2nd little carrots
- 2 sticks celery
- 1 onion
- 1 clove of garlic
- 2 tbsp oil Salt Pepper
- 850 g canned tomatoes
- 200 ml exemplary vegetable stock
- 1 tsp fennel seeds
- 30 g parmesan (1 piece)
- Nutmeg
- 225 g ricotta
- 16 entire grain lasagna sheets
- Butter for the form
- 150 g mozzarella

Let the spinach defrost. Hack the seitan finely or put it through the center cut of the meat processor.

Wash and strip carrots. Wash, clean, expel, and finely dice the celery. Strip and cleave the onion and garlic.

Heat the oil during a pan and braise the carrots, celery, onions, and garlic for 3 minutes over medium warmth. Include from that point forward and braise for 3 minutes while mixing. Season with salt and pepper.

Put the canned tomatoes and stock within the pan and spread and cook over medium warmth for 20 minutes, mixing every so often. Pulverize the fennel seeds, include, and season the sauce with salt and pepper.

Meanwhile, finely grind the Parmesan. Concentrate on some nutmeg. Crush the spinach enthusiastically, generally slash, and blend during a bowl with the ricotta, parmesan, salt, pepper, and nutmeg.

Lightly oil a preparing dish (approx. 30 x 20 cm). Spread rock bottom of the shape with slightly sauce and smooth it out. Spot 4 sheets of lasagna on the brink of every other, if essential slice to estimate. Add 1/3 of the spinach blend and smooth. Spread 1/4 of the sauce on top. Layer 4 lasagna sheets, 1/3 spinach, and 1/4 sauce once more, rehash the procedure. Place the keep going lasagna sheets on top and spread the remainder of the sauce over them.

Drain the mozzarella and attack enormous pieces. Spread on the lasagna. Heat veggie-lover lasagna during a preheated stove at 180 ° C (fan broiler: 160 ° C, gas: levels 2–3) on the center rack for 35–40 minutes. Let the veggie lover lasagna rest for around 5 minutes before serving.

241. Asparagus and Ham Omelet with Potatoes and Parsley

- 200 g new potatoes
- Salt
- 150 g white asparagus
- 1 onion
- 50 g bresaola (Italian meat ham)
- 2 stems parsley
- 3 eggs
- 1 tbsp rapeseed oil
- Pepper

Wash the potatoes well. Cook in bubbling salted water for approx. 20 minutes, channel and let cool. While the potatoes are cooking, strip the asparagus, remove the lower woody closures. Cook asparagus in salted water for around quarter-hour, scoop of the water, channel well and let cool. Strip the onion and hack finely.

Cut the asparagus and potatoes into little pieces.

Cut the bresaola into strips.

Wash parsley, shake dry, pluck leaves, and slash. Beat the eggs during a bowl and race with the hacked parsley.

Heat the oil during a covered skillet and sauté the onion solid shapes until medium-high warmth until translucent.

Add potatoes and keep it up simmering for 2 minutes.

Add asparagus and fry for 1 moment.

Add the bresaola and season everything with salt and pepper. Put the eggs within the skillet and spread and stew for 5–6 minutes over low warmth. Drop out of the skillet and serve directly.

242. Poached Eggs on Spinach with sauce

- 1 clove of garlic
- 3 tsp. oil
- 1 tsp. sugar
- 200 ml wine
- Salt
- Pepper
- 1 shallot
- 250 g youthful spinach leaves
- Nutmeg
- 2 tbsp vinegar
- 4 eggs
- 2 cuts entire grain toast

Peel and finely slash the garlic and braise in 1 teaspoon of oil. Sprinkle sugar, include wine, and convey to the bubble. Lessen to 1/3 over medium warmth. Salt, pepper and keep warm.

Peel the shallot and shakers finely. Wash the spinach well and let it channel. Warmth the rest of the oil during a skillet, sauté the shallot during a smooth warmth. Include the spinach and let it a breakdown in 3-4 minutes. Include slightly nutmeg, salt, and pepper.

Boil 1 liter of water with the vinegar. Painstakingly beat the eggs during a bowl with the goal that the yolks stay flawless. Stir the bubbling vinegar water energetically with a whisk.

Now let the eggs slide in (by the pivot of the water they separate right away). Boil the water once more. Expel the pot from the hob at that point and allow the eggs to cook for 3-4 minutes (poach).

Scoop the eggs with a froth trowel and permit them to channel. Put the spinach on a plate and put the eggs thereon. Shower with the sauce and serve. Toast the bread within the toaster and present with it.

243. Pasta with Minced Lamb Balls and Eggplant, Tomatoes and Sultanas

- 250 gleans minced sheep
- 2 tbsp low-fat quark
- 1 egg
- 2 tbsp breadcrumbs
- Salt
- Pepper
- 1 tsp. cinnamon
- 200 g little eggplant (1 little eggplant)
- 1 onion
- 1 clove of garlic
- 2 tbsp oil
- 150 g orecchiette pasta
- 2 tbsp sultanas
- 400 g pizza tomatoes (can)
- 1 straight leaf
- 125 ml great vegetable stock

Mix minced sheep, quark, egg, and breadcrumbs during a bowl. Season with salt, pepper, and cinnamon.

Using wet hands, transform the slash into balls the size of a cherry. Chill quickly.

Clean, wash, dry the eggplant, and dig 5 mm blocks. Strip onion and garlic and hack finely.

Heat 1 tablespoon of oil during a skillet and fry the meatballs in it until brilliant earthy colored. Expel and put during a secure spot.

Wipe out the dish and afterward heat up the rest of the oil. Include the eggplant shapes, onion, and garlic and braise for 4-5 minutes, mixing. Meanwhile, cook the pasta nibble verification during tons of bubbling salted water as per the bundle guidelines.

Add the sultanas, tomatoes, and sound leave to the skillet. Pour within the stock and convey it to the bubble.

Cover and cook for 4 minutes over medium warmth. At that point put the meatballs within the dish and cook secured for an extra 5

244. Vegetable Spaghetti

- 200 g red chime pepper (1 red ringer pepper)
- 200 g yellow chime pepper (1 yellow ringer pepper)
- 150 g carrots (2 carrots)
- 300 g broccoli
- 12 yellow cherry tomatoes
- ½ pack parsley
- 20 g tawny (8 leaves)
- 3 spring onions
- 300 g entire grain spaghetti
- Salt
- ½ lemon
- 4 tbsp oil Pepper

Quarter the peppers, center them, wash and spot them on a heating sheet, skin side up. Broil under the recent flame broil until the skin turns dark and rankles.

Cover and let cool during a bowl secured for 10 minutes (steam). At that point skin and dig fine strips.

Peel the carrots and cut them into flimsy cuts.

Clean broccoli, dig little florets and wash. Wash and split tomatoes.

Clean the parsley, shake it out, pick up the leaves, clean and wash roan, generally hack both. The spring onions are cleaned, washed and cut into meager cuts.

Cook the spaghetti nibble evidence during tons of salted water as indicated by the bundle directions. Include broccoli and carrots 4 minutes before the finish of the cooking time. Squeeze lemon. Channel the pasta and blend during a bowl with the readied Ingredients:, 1 teaspoon lemon squeeze, and oil.

245. Spaghetti with Salmon in Lemon Sauce

- 150 g salmon filet (without skin)
- 100 g leek (1 flimsy stick)
- 100 g little carrots (2 little carrots)
- ½ natural lemon
- 2 stems parsley
- 150 g entire grain spaghetti Salt
- 2 tbsp oil Pepper
- 100 ml of fish stock
- 150 ml of soy cream

Wash salmon, pat dry, and dig 2 cm 3D squares.

The leek is dried, washed and cut into dainty circles. Strip the carrots and cut them into flimsy strips.

Within the interim, wash the lemon half hot and rub dry. Strip the lemon strip meagerly and dig fine strips. Crush juice. Wash parsley, shake dry, pluck leaves and cleave finely. Cook the pasta chomp verification in saltwater as indicated by the bundle guidelines.

Heat oil during a dish. Season the salmon with pepper and fry everywhere within the recent oil for 3-4 minutes.

Remove the salmon, braise the leek rings, and carrot strips within the dish over medium warmth for 3-4 minutes.

Remove the salmon, braise the leek rings, and carrot strips within the dish over medium warmth for 3-4 minutes.

If fundamental, salt the salmon, set it back within the container, and warmth quickly. Blend within the parsley. Drain the pasta during a strainer and blend tenderly with the sauce. Season with salt and pepper and directly serve the spaghetti and salmon.

246. Kale and red onion dahl with Buckwheat

- one tablespoon olive oil
- One very little very little onion sliced
- Two cm ginger grated
- One eye chilli deseeded and finely cleaved (more on the off likelihood that you just that you just things hot!)
- two teaspoons turmeric
- Two teaspoons garam masala
- One hundred sixty g very little lentils
- four hundred cc cc milk
- two hundred cc cc
- A hundred g kale or spinach would be a unprecedented unprecedented One hundred sixty g buckwheat or brown rice

Place the olive oil in a very vast, deep saucepan and embody the cut onion.

Cook on a low heat, with the lid on for 5.

Add the garlic, ginger and chilli and cook for one more minute.

Add the turmeric, garam masala and a splash of water and cook for one a lot of a lot of.

Add the red lentils, coconut milk, and 200ml water (do this simply by half filling embody coconut milk can with water and tipping it into the saucepan). Combine everything together altogether and embody for twenty 5 associate degree a twenty heat with the cover cover. Stir once throughout a jiffy and embody water if the dhal starts to stick.

After twenty minutes add the kale, stir thoroughly and replace the cover, embody for a further five 5 7. About fifteen ready, place embody buckwheat in a medium pot and add plenty of effervescent water. Bring the water back dahl the boil and cook for ten minutes

247. Buckwheat food Salad-Sirt Food Recipes

- 50g buckwheat pasta (cooked according to the packet guidelines) Large handful of rocket
- Small bunch of basil leaves
- Eight cherry tomatoes, halved
- 1/2 avocado, diced
- Ten olives
- one tbsp extra virgin edible fat
- 20g pine loco

Gently combine all the ingredients except the pine nuts and arrange on a plate or in a bowl, then scatter the pine nuts over the top.

248. Greek dish Skewers

306 Calories, 3.5 of your SIRT five a day, Serves 2 Ready place 10 5

- Two wood wood, soaked in water cookery 30 minutes before use
- Eight vast dark olives
- Eight cherry tomatoes
- One yellow pepper, cut into eight squares
- ½ red onion hamper the middle the middle into eight items 100g (about 10cm) cucumber, dig four cuts and halved 100g feta, cut into eight cubes
- For the dressing:
- one tbsp to boot further olive oil associate degree of ½ half One tsp oleoresin vinegar
- ½ clove garlic, peeled and press
- Few leaves basil, finely chopped (or ½ tsp dried mingling to replace basil and oregano)
- Few leaves oregano, finely hacked
- Generous seasoning of salt and freshly ground dark pepper

Thread each skewer with the salad Ingredients: place the order: olive, tomato, yellow pepper, red onion, cucumber, feta, tomato, olive, yellow pepper, red onion, cucumber, and feta.

Place all the dressing Ingredients: place a small bowl and mix together thoroughly. Pour associate degree the sticks.

249. Kale, Edamame and curd Curry-Sirt Food Recipes

- One tbsp oilseed oil
- One large onion, hacked
- Four garlic, stripped and three
- One vast thumb (7cm) new ginger, peeled and ground One red stew, deseeded and thinly sliced 1/2 tsp ground turmeric
- 1/4 tsp cayenne pepper
- One tsp paprika
- 1/2 one ground cumin

- one tsp salt
- 250g dried two lentils
- One litre boiling water
- 50g frozen soyaedamame beans
- 200g firm tofu, hacked into cubes
- Two tomatoes, roughly hacked
- Juice of one embody
- 200g kale leaves, stalks expelled and torn

Place the oil place associate degree associate degree associate degree associate degree a low-medium heat. Embody the embody and embody for 5 5 5 5 the three, ginger and stew and preparation preparation a preparation two preparation. Embody the turmeric, cayenne, paprika, cumin and salt. Stir through 5 5 the red lentils and stirring once more.

Pour in the boiling water and bring Cajanus cajan a hearty simmer for ten minutes, then reduce the heat and cook for a further 20-30 minutes till the curry options an options options consistency.

Add the soya beans, bean curd and tomatoes and cook preparation a preparation five preparation. Embody embody embody juice and kale leaves and cook till embody kale is just tender.

250. Sirt Food Miso Marinated Cod with herb

Serves 1

- 20g miso
- One tbsp mirin
- One tbsp extra virgin olive oil
- 200g skinless cod filet
- 20g two onion, sliced
- 40g celery, sliced
- One garlic clove, finely chopped
- One bird's eye bean stew, finely chopped One one finely slashed new ginger 60g inexperienced beans
- 50g kale, typically chopped
- One tsp herb herb
- 5g parsley, typically chopped
- one tbsp tamari
- 30g buckwheat
- one tsp ground turmeric

Mix the miso, mirin and one teaspoon two the oil. Rub all over the cod and leave to marinate for thirty thirty. Heat the oven Cajanus cajan 220ºC/gas seven.

Bake the cod preparation ten preparation.

Meanwhile, heat an associate degree cooking pan or cooking pan with embody cooking pan oil. Embody the onion and pan deep- fried food for a number of of moments, then add the celery, garlic, chilli, ginger, green beans and kale. Toss and fry 5 the kale is tender and grilled grilled. You may need to include slightly to help to help process.

Cook the buckwheat according to the bundle instructions with the turmeric for three 5.

Add the sesame seeds, parsley and tamari to embody pan sear and serve with embody greens and fish.

251. Beef bourguignon with Mashed Potatoes and Kale

Preparation time: 15 minutes. - **Cooking time:** 2–3 hours. - **Serving:** 4

- 800 grams diced beef

- 1 tablespoon extra-virgin olive oil
- 150 grams red onion, roughly chopped
- 200 grams celery, roughly chopped
- 100 grams carrots, roughly chopped
- 2–3 cloves of garlic, chopped
- 375 milliliters of red wine
- 2 tablespoon tomato puree
- 750 milliliters beef broth
- 2 bay leaves
- 1 sprig of fresh thyme or 1 tablespoon of dried thyme
- 75 grams diced pancetta or smoked lard
- 250 grams mushrooms
- 2 tablespoon chopped parsley
- 200 grams kale
- 1 tablespoon cornflour or arrowroot (optional)

For the porridge:
- 500 grams Edward potatoes
- 1 tablespoon milk and 1 tablespoon olive oil

1. Pat the beef dry with kitchen paper. Heat a heavy saucepan over medium-high heat. Add the olive oil, then the beef and saute the meat until completely browned. Depending on the size of your pan, it's best to do this in 3– 4 small loads.

2. When all of the meat is brown, remove it from the pan with a slotted spoon and set aside. Add the onion, celery, carrot and garlic to the same pan and fry for 3 to 4 minutes over medium heat until tender. Add the wine, tomato paste and broth and bring to a boil. Add the browned beef, bay leaves and thyme and reduce the heat to a simmer. Cover the pan with a lid and cook for 2 hours to ensure that nothing sticks to the rim, stirring from time to time. While the beef is cooking, peel your potatoes and cut them into quarters (or smaller pieces if they're quite large).

3. Put in a pan with cold water and bring to a boil. Reduce the heat to a simmer and cook for 20–25 minutes, covered with a lid. When soft, drain and mash with olive oil and milk. Keep warm. While the potatoes are boiling, heat a pan over high heat. Then add the diced pancetta when it's hot but not smoking.

4. The fat content of the bacon means you don't need oil to cook it. Once some of the fat is released and it begins to brown, add the mushrooms and cook over medium heat until both are nicely browned. Depending on the size of your pan, you may need to do this in multiple loads. Set aside after cooking. Cook or steam the kale for 5–10 minutes until soft. Once the beef is tender enough and the sauce has thickened to your liking, add the pancetta, mushrooms, and parsley. If your sauce is always kind of runny, you can mix the cornflour or arrowroot with a little water and then stir the paste into the sauce until you have the consistency you want. Cook for 2-3 minutes and serve with porridge and kale.

Nutrition Carbohydrates: 34g **Fat:** 25g **Protein:** 31g **Kcal:** 510cal

252. Turkish fajitas

Preparation time: 15 minutes. - **Cooking time:** approx. 1 hour. - **Serving:** 4

For the filling:
- 500 grams turkey breast into strips
- 1 tablespoon of extra virgin olive oil 1–2 chilies, depending on taste, chopped
- 150 grams red onion, thinly sliced
- 150 grams red pepper, cut into thin strips 2–3 cloves of garlic, chopped

- 1 tablespoon paprika
- 1 tablespoon ground cumin
- 1 teaspoon chili powder
- 1 tablespoon chopped coriander

For the guacamole:
- 2 ripe avocados, peeled (reserve one of the stones)
- Juice of 1 lime
- Pinch of chili powder
- Pinch of black pepper

For the salsa:
- 1×400 grams can of chopped tomatoes 20 grams red onion, diced
- 20 grams red pepper, deseeded and diced Juice of ½–1 lime, depending on the size 1 teaspoon chopped coriander
- 1 teaspoon capers

For the salad:
- 100 grams rocket
- 3 tomatoes, cut
- 100 grams cucumber, thinly sliced
- 1 tablespoon extra-virgin olive oil juice of ½ lemon

For serving:
- 100 grams cheddar cheese
- 8 grated whole grain tortilla wraps

1. Mix together the filling ingredients and set them aside while the other parts are prepared.

2. In a small food processor, bring all the guacamole ingredients in and flash until a smooth paste is formed. Alternatively, you can mash them all together with the back of a fork or spoon.

3. Place the reserved avocado stone in the guacamole—it will keep it from turning brown. Mix all the ingredients for the salsa.

4. Put all the salad ingredients in a large tub. Put your largest pan on high heat until it starts to smoke.

5. Put the turkey filling in the hot pan - you may need to cook it in 2 to 3 loads as overcrowding the pan will create too much moisture and it will start boiling instead of frying.

6. Keep the pan over high heat and keep moving the mixture, so the turkey colors nicely but doesn't burn.

7. In a low oven, keep the cooked meat warm. To serve, reheat the tortillas according to the directions in the package, then sprinkle some guacamole over each package.

8. Top with some cheese and some salsa, then stack the turkey mixture in the middle and roll it up like a large cigar. Serve with the salad.

Nutrition Carbohydrates: 44g **Fat:** 21g **Protein:** 30g **Kcal:** 450cal

253. Sirt Chicken Korma

Preparation time: 10 minutes - Cooking time: 50 minutes - Serving: 4
- 350 ml chicken stock
- 30 g Medjool date, chopped
- 2 cinnamon sticks
- 4–5 cardamom pods, slightly split 250 ml coconut milk
- 8 boneless, skinless chicken thighs
- 1 tablespoon ground turmeric
- 200 g buckwheat
- 150 ml of Greek yogurt
- 50 g of ground walnuts
- 2 tablespoon chopped coriander

For the curry paste

- 1 large red onion, quartered
- 3 cloves of garlic
- 2 cm piece of fresh ginger
- 1 tbsp mild curry powder
- 1 teaspoon ground cumin
- 1 tbsp ground turmeric
- 1 tbsp coconut oil

1. In a food processor, place the ingredients for the curry paste and flash for about a minute until you have a nice paste.
2. Alternatively, you can use a pestle and mortar to grind it. Fry the paste in a heavy pan over medium heat for 1-2 minutes then add the broth, date, cinnamon, cardamom pods, and coconut milk.
3. Bring to a boil then add the chicken legs. Reduce the heat, cover the pan with a lid, and simmer for 45 minutes.
4. Meanwhile, bring it to a boil with a pan of water and whisk in the turmeric.
5. Add the buckwheat and cook according to the directions on the package. As soon as the chicken is tender, stir in the yogurt and cook the walnuts over low heat for a few more minutes.
6. Add the coriander and serve with the buckwheat

Nutrition Carbohydrates: 21 **Fat**: 16 **Protein**: 32 **Kcal**: 330

254. *Prawns, Pak Choi and broccoli*

Preparation time: 15 minutes - Cooking time: 20 minutes - Serving: 5

- 1 tbsp ground turmeric
- 400 g raw shrimp, peeled and deveined
- 1 tbsp coconut oil
- 280 g buckwheat noodles
- 1 teaspoon virgin olive oil
- For the china pan
- 1 tbsp coconut oil
- Cut 250 g broccoli into bite-sized pieces 250 g pak choi, roughly chopped 1 red onion, thinly sliced
- 2 cm piece of fresh ginger, chopped 1–2 chili peppers, chopped
- 3 cloves of garlic, chopped
- 150 ml vegetable broth
- 1 bunch of basil, removed leaves and chopped stems
- 1 tbsp Thai fish sauce or tamari

Mix the turmeric with the prawns. Place the coconut oil in a wok or pan and cook the shrimp over medium-high heat for a time of 3 to 4 minutes or until it is opaque.
After cooking, remove from pan and set aside. Wipe the pan for the pan and put it on high heat until it starts to smoke.
Add the coconut oil then add the vegetables, ginger, chili peppers, and garlic.
Keep moving the vegetables in the pan so they don't burn. Cook for 3–5 minutes - lower the heat a little if the vegetables look charred - until they are fried but crispy.
Add the broth, whole basil and fish sauce.
Bring to the boil, then add the shrimp and let heat. In the meantime, cook the pasta according to the instructions on the package.
Freshen up in cold water and mix with the olive oil to prevent them from sticking together. Serve the pan with the hot noodles.

Nutrition Carbohydrates: 13 Fat: 15 Protein: 26 Kcal: 270

255. *Cocoa spaghetti Bolognese*

Preparation time: 15 minutes - Cooking time: approx. 1 hour - Serving: 4

- 1 tbsp virgin olive oil
- 1 red onion, finely diced
- 100 g celery, finely diced
- 100 g carrots, finely diced
- 3 cloves of garlic, chopped
- 400 g of lean ground beef
- 1 tbsp Herbs de Provence
- 1–2 bay leaves
- 150 ml red wine
- 300 ml beef broth
- 1 tbsp cocoa powder
- 1 tbsp tomato paste
- 2 × 400 g cans of chopped tomatoes
- 280 g whole wheat spaghetti
- 1 teaspoon ground black pepper
- 1 bunch of fresh basil
- 20 g parmesan cheese

Heat the oil in a pan and then cook the onion, celery, carrot and garlic over medium heat for 1-2 minutes until they are a little softer.
Add the ground beef and dried herbs and cook over medium-high heat until the ground beef is brown.
Add the wine, stock, cocoa powder, tomato paste and canned tomatoes, bring to a boil and simmer for 45 to 60 minutes with the lid closed.
When you're almost done, cook the pasta as directed on the package.
Finally stir the pepper and basil leaves into the sauce. Serve with the pasta and rub some parmesan on top.

Nutrition Carbohydrates: 43 Fat: 21m Protein: 11 Kcal: 450

256. *Baked salmon with Watercress sauce and Potatoes*

Preparation time: 10 minutes - Cooking time: 35 minutes - Serving: 4

- 400 g of new potatoes
- 4 × 125 g skinless salmon fillets
- 1 teaspoon extra virgin olive oil
- 1 piece of broccoli, cut into florets
- 1 bunch of asparagus spears

For the watercress sauce
- 30 g of watercress
- 5 g parsley
- 1 tbsp capers
- 2 tbsp virgin olive oil
- Extra juice of 1 lemon

Heat the oven to 200 ° C / gas. 6. Place the potatoes with cold water in a tub.
Bring to a boil and simmer for 15-20 minutes or until tender.
Brush the olive oil with the salmon fillets, put them on a baking sheet and bake for 10 minutes in the oven.
When you like your salmon to be lightly cooked, reduce the cooking time by 2 to 3 minutes.
In the meantime, cook or steam the broccoli and asparagus until tender.
Put the ingredients for the sauce in a food processor or blender and stir until smooth. Serve the salmon with the sauce and the vegetables.

Nutrition Carbohydrates: 9 Fat: 15 Protein: 31 Kcal: 250

257. Coq au vin with potatoes and green beans

Preparation time: 10 minutes- Cooking time: 35 minutes - Serving: 4

- 4 skinless chicken legs
- 4 skinless chicken legs
- 1-2 tbsp buckwheat flour
- 1 tbsp extra virgin olive oil
- 150 g red onion
- 150 g carrot
- 200 g celery
- 3 cloves of garlic, chopped
- 400 ml red wine
- 400 ml of chicken broth
- 1 sprig of fresh thyme
- 2–3 bay leaves
- 100 g pancetta or smoked bacon, diced
- 250 g mushrooms
- 400 g of new potatoes
- 2 tbsp chopped parsley
- 250 g green beans

Roll the chicken pieces in the flour. Heat a heavy saucepan over medium-high heat. Then add the olive oil and the chicken and cook until all is nicely browned.

Remove and set aside from the pan. Add the onion, carrot, celery and garlic to the same pan and cook gently for 2-3 minutes until softened.

When the pan is dry, you can add some water here. Add the wine and chicken stock and bring to a boil. Add the thyme, bay leaves, and chicken. Cover and simmer gently for 45 minutes with a lid.

Check the amount of fluid from time to time and add a little more. Heat a pan over high heat. Then add the diced pancetta when it's hot but not smoking.

Once some of the fat is released and it begins to brown, add the mushrooms and cook over medium heat until both it and the pancetta are nicely browned.

Depending on the size of your pan, you may need to do this in multiple loads. Set aside after cooking.

Using cold water to place the potatoes in a tub. Bring to a boil and simmer for 15-20 minutes or until tender. When you're done, drain it and return to the pan to keep it warm.

Add the pancetta, mushrooms and parsley to the Coq au Vin and cook for another 15 minutes.

To cook the green beans, steam them or cook them for 4 to 6 minutes, depending on how crispy you like them.

With the potatoes and beans, serve the Coq au Vin.

Nutrition Carbohydrates: 13 Fat: 15 Protein: 26 Kcal: 270

258. Salmon buckwheat Pasta

Preparation time: 10 minutes - Cooking time: 25 minutes - Serving: 4

- 300 g skinless salmon fillet
- 1 teaspoon extra virgin olive oil
- 250 g buckwheat noodles
- 100 g kale, chopped
- 1 large zucchini, quarter lengthways
- Cut 1 red onion into slices
- Cut 4 cloves of garlic into slices
- 1 tbsp Herbs of Provence
- 1 tbsp extra virgin olive oil

For the sauce
- 650 ml milk or dairy-free alternative
- 65 g unsalted butter
- 65 g buckwheat or flour
- 150 g cheddar cheese, grated
- 2 tbsp chopped parsley
- 2 tbsp capers

Heat the oven to 200 ° C / gas. 6. Rub the salmon with olive oil and put it on a piece of foil.

Fold over the edges and seal them to get a package. Bake in the oven for 15 minutes.

Cook the pasta on the box according to the instructions. Drain, then pour some warm water out of the kettle to prevent it from sticking and put aside.

To make the sauce, bring the milk to a boil in a small saucepan, being careful not to overflow it.

Then melt the butter and add it to a separate pan. Mix them together until you have a mixture.

Cook gently over low heat for 30 seconds to 1 minute. Gradually add the hot milk, stirring continuously, until you have a nice thick sauce.

Add 100 g cheese, parsley and capers and remove from heat. In the meantime, cook or steam the kale until tender.

Cook the zucchini in a pan over medium heat, red onion, garlic and herbs in the olive oil for 2-3 minutes until tender. Mix with the cooked kale.

Heat a grill on the highest setting. Peel the cooked salmon and mix with the pasta, cooked vegetables and sauce, place in an ovenproof bowl and sprinkle over the remaining cheese.

Place under the hot grill for 5 minutes until the cheese turns brown.

Nutrition Carbohydrates: 13 Fat: 15 Protein: 26 Kcal: 270

259. Cauliflower Kale curry

Preparation time: 10 minutes - Cooking time: 30 minutes - Serving: 4

- 200 g buckwheat
- 2 tbsp ground turmeric
- 1 red onion, chopped
- 3 cloves of garlic, minced
- 2.5 cm piece of fresh ginger, chopped
- 1–2 chili peppers, chopped
- 1 tbsp coconut oil
- 1 tbsp mild curry powder
- 1 tbsp ground cumin
- 2 × 400 g cans of chopped tomatoes
- 300 ml vegetable broth
- 200 g kale, roughly chopped
- 300 g cauliflower, chopped
- 1 × 400 g can of butter beans, drained
- 2 tomatoes, cut into wedges
- 2 tbsp chopped coriander

Cook the buckwheat and add 1 tablespoon of turmeric to the water, as per the directions on the package.

In the meantime, cook the onion, garlic, ginger and chili peppers in the coconut oil over medium heat for 2-3 minutes. Add the seasonings, including the remaining tablespoon of turmeric and continue cooking over low to medium heat for 1–2 minutes.

Add the canned tomatoes and the broth and bring to a boil then simmer for 10 minutes.

Add the kale, cauliflower and butter beans and cook for 10 minutes.

Add the tomato wedges and coriander and cook for another minute.

Then serve them with the buckwheat.

Nutrition Carbohydrates: 43 Fat: 21 Protein: 11 Kcal: 450

260. Kidney bean burritos

Preparation time: 15 minutes - Cooking time: 45 minutes - Serving: 4

- 1 tbsp extra virgin olive oil
- 1 red onion, diced
- 3 cloves of garlic, chopped
- 1 tablespoon chili, chopped
- 1 tbsp paprika
- 1 tbsp ground cumin
- 1 teaspoon chili powder
- 1 tbsp chopped coriander
- 2 tomatoes, chopped
- 3 × 400 g cans of kidney beans, drained
- 500 ml vegetable broth
- 150 g cheddar or vegan cheese
- 8 whole grain tortilla wraps
- 1 × 500 g glass of tomato passata
- 1 × 200 g jar of jalepeño peppers (optional)

For the salad:

- 125 g rocket
- 1 paprika,
- 3 tomatoes sliced,
- ½ small red onion sliced
- 1 avocado cut into slices, peeled and sliced
- 1 tablespoon of extra virgin olive oil juice ½ lemon

Heat a large saucepan over medium heat. Apply the olive oil and sauté for 1-2 minutes with the onion, garlic and chili, until slightly softer.

Add the coriander and spices and cook for another 1–2 minutes. Add the tomatoes, kidney beans and broth. Bring to a boil and cook over medium-high heat for 20 minutes.

You want most of the liquid to evaporate. So keep an eye out for them and stir sometimes.

Take off the stove and let cool down a bit. Take about a third of the kidney beans out of the pan and set aside. In a food processor or blender, soften the remaining mixture, then return to the pan, add the whole beans and stir in.

The mixture should be a little stiff. Allowing it to cool fully would make wrapping the burritos easier. Heat the oven to 200 ° C / gas. 6th

Spread the cheese on top of the wraps, holding back a little to spread over the top at the end. Divide the filling and roll each into a sausage tin between the wraps.

Spread a thin layer of passata on the bottom of an ovenproof bowl large enough to hold all of the burritos in a single layer.

Put them in this way and drizzle the rest of the passata over them.

Sprinkle with the remaining cheese and the jalepeños, if used.

Cover the bowl with foil and bake in the oven for 20-25 minutes. Remove the foil and bake for another 5 minutes to brown the cheese.

Throw all the salad ingredients together and serve with the hot burritos.

Nutrition Carbohydrates: 43 Fat: 21 Protein: 11 Kcal: 450

261. Spiced Cauliflower Couscous with Chicken

Preparation time: 15 minutes - **Cooking time:** 20 minutes - **Servings**: 2

- 2 cups roughly chopped cauliflower florets
- A handful fresh flat-leaf parsley
- 2 cloves garlic, finely chopped
- ½ cup finely chopped red onions
- 2 teaspoons finely chopped ginger
- 1/3 cup sun-dried tomatoes
- 2 tablespoons capers
- 2 chicken breasts
- 4 teaspoons turmeric powder
- ½ cup finely diced carrots
- 2 bird's eye chilies, finely chopped
- 4 tablespoons extra-virgin olive oil
- Juice of a lemon

1. You can chop the cauliflower in a food processor.
2. Place a pan over medium – high flame. Add 2 tablespoons oil. When the oil is warmed, add the ginger, the garlic and the chili and cook until fragrant for a few seconds.
3. Stir in turmeric and cook for 5 – 8 seconds. Stir in the carrots and cauliflower and cook for about 2 minutes. Turn off the heat.
4. Transfer into a bowl. Add tomatoes and parsley and stir. Keep warm.
5. Add remaining oil into the pan and let it heat. Place chicken in the pan and cook for about 6 minutes. Turn over the chicken and cook for 5 to 6 minutes or until the inside is well-cooked.
6. Stir in capers, lemon juice and a sprinkle of water.
7. Add cauliflower and carrot mixture and toss well.

Nutrition: Calories: 250 Fat: 4.5g Protein: 68g Total Carbohydrates: 13g Dietary Fiber: 5g Sodium: 532mg

262. Chicken Noodles

Preparation time: 10 minutes - **Cooking time**: 30 minutes - **Servings**: 8 – 10

- 16 ounces buckwheat noodles
- 2 yellow bell peppers, chopped into ½ inch squares
- 6 cloves garlic, chopped
- 2 tablespoons olive oil
- 6 cups tomato sauce
- 2 tablespoons fresh basil, chopped or 2 teaspoons dry basil
- 2 tablespoons fresh parsley, chopped or 2 teaspoons dried parsley
- Pepper to taste
- 2 pounds skinless, boneless chicken breast, cut into strips
- 1 large red onion, chopped into ½ inch squares, separate the layers
- Salt to taste

1. On the box, follow the instructions and cook the buckwheat noodles.
2. Place a large skillet over medium flame. Add the oil and wait until the oil is hot. Add chicken strips and spread it all over the pan and cook undisturbed, until the underside is cooked. Flip sides and cook the other side, undisturbed.
3. Add the vegetables and mix well. Cook until the vegetables are tender. Add tomato sauce and cook for 7-8 minutes.
4. Add noodles and toss well.

Nutrition: Calories 372.3 Total Fat 12.4 g Protein 42.6 g Carbs 26.1 g

263. Chicken Butternut Squash Pasta

Preparation time: 10 minutes - **Cooking time:** 30 – 40 minutes - **Servings:** 2

- ½ pound ground chicken
- tablespoon balsamic vinegar
- ½ tablespoon olive oil, divided
- ½ cups whole wheat pasta
- Pepper to taste
- fresh basil leaves, thinly sliced
- tablespoons chopped walnuts
- Salt to taste
- ½ cups cubed butternut squash, cut into ½" cubes
- ounces goat's cheese, crumbled
- ½ teaspoon garlic, minced
- 1/8 teaspoon ground nutmeg

1 Place butternut squash on a baking sheet. Drizzle 1 tablespoon oil and sprinkle salt and pepper over the squash. Toss well.

2 Bake squash in an oven preheated to 400° F, for about 30 minutes or until tender.

3 Following the package instructions, cook the pasta.

4 Place a skillet over medium heat. Add ½ tablespoon oil and wait for it to heat. Add garlic and cook until light brown, stirring often.

5 Attach the chicken and simmer until the chicken is no longer pink.

6 Stir in walnuts, nutmeg and vinegar.

7 Cook on low heat for 1 – 2 minutes.

8 Serve chicken over pasta.

9 Scatter butternut squash and goat's cheese. Sprinkle basil on top.

Nutrition: Sodium: 198 mg Cholesterol: 0.0 mg Total Carbs: 39.0 g Fiber:15.0 g Protein: 12.0 g Calories: 247.0

264. Chicken Marsala

Preparation time: 10 minutes - **Cooking time:** 30 – 40 minutes - **Servings:** 8

- 8 boneless, skinless breasts of chicken (6 ounces each)
- 20 ounces cremini mushrooms, sliced
- 2 cloves garlic, peeled, sliced
- 1 cup marsala wine
- 6 tablespoons flour
- 2 large shallots, chopped
- Salt to taste
- 1 cup chicken broth
- Freshly ground pepper to taste
- 4 – 5 tablespoons olive oil
- 2 tablespoons chopped parsley
- Sautéed spinach to serve

1. Place the chicken breasts between 2 sheets of plastic wrap and pound them with a meat mallet until ½ inch thick.

2. Sprinkle salt and pepper over the chicken. Sprinkle flour over the chicken.

3. Place a large skillet over medium flame. To spread the oil, add about a tablespoon of oil and swirl in the pan.

4. In the pan, put as many pieces of chicken as possible. Sear the chicken on both the sides until golden brown. Remove the chicken from the pan placed on a plate using a slotted spoon.

5. In the same way, cook the remaining chicken, adding more oil if needed.

6. Add 2 tablespoons oil into the skillet. When the oil is heated, add mushrooms and cook until brown.

7. Stir in garlic and shallots. Stir-fry for 1 and add salt and pepper to taste. – 2 minutes.

8. Add wine, broth and chicken along with the released juice and cook until the liquid in the pan is half its original quantity.

9. Garnish with parsley and serve along with sautéed spinach or any other sautéed greens of your choice.

Nutrition: Calories: 90 Sodium: 20mg Fat: 3g Cholesterol: 2mg Carbohydrates: 11g Protein: 3g

265. Turkey Apple Burgers

Preparation time: 15 minutes - **Cooking time:** 8 – 10 minutes - **Servings:** 2

- 1 green apple, cored, peeled, halved
- A handful fresh thyme or sage, minced
- Pepper to taste
- ½ teaspoon onion powder
- ¼ teaspoon garlic powder
- Salt to taste
- 1 teaspoon olive oil
- ½ pound 93% lean ground turkey
- Whole-wheat burger buns or lettuce cups to serve

1. Grate one half of the apple and cut the other half into thin slices.

2. Combine grated apple, spices, salt, sage and turkey in a bowl and mix well.

3. Make 2 equal portions of the mixture. Shape into patties.

4. Place a skillet over medium flame. Brush both sides of the patties with oil and put in the tub.

5. Cook until the underside is brown. Turn the burgers over and cook the other side until brown.

6. Serve burgers over buns or lettuce cups. Place sliced apples on top of the burgers and serve.

Nutrition: Calories: 10 218 215 Total Fat: 15 613 Saturated Fat: 3753 Sodium: 1342 Total Carbohydrate: Protein: 121

266. Turkey Sandwiches with Apple and Walnut Mayo

Preparation time: 15 minutes - **Cooking time:** 4 minutes - **Servings:** 2

For walnut mayonnaise:

- 2 tablespoons finely chopped walnuts
- 3 – 4 tablespoons mayonnaise
- ½ tablespoon Dijon mustard
- ½ tablespoon chopped, fresh parsley

For sandwich:

- 4 slices whole-wheat bread
- ½ green apple, peeled, cored, cut into thin slices
- Cooked, sliced turkey, as required
- A handful rockets

1. To make walnut mayonnaise: Combine walnuts, mayonnaise, mustard and parsley in a bowl.

2. Smear walnut mayonnaise on one side of the bread slices.

3. Place arugula on 2 bread slices, on the mayo side. Place turkey slices over it followed by apple slices.

4. Complete the sandwich by covering with remaining bread slices, with mayo side facing down.

5. Cut into desired shape and serve.

Nutrition: Calories: 205 Protein: 5.2g Carbs: 30.7g Fat: 12.1g Sodium: 66. 5mg

267. Sautéed Turkey with Tomatoes and Cilantro

Preparation time: 10 minutes - **Cooking time**: 15 minutes - **Servings**: 2 – 3
- ½ pound lean ground turkey
- ½ cup chopped yellow or red onion
- Pepper to taste
- 1 teaspoon olive oil
- 1 jalapeño or to taste, chopped
- ½ tablespoon minced garlic
- ¼ cup chopped tomatoes
- ¼ teaspoon ground cumin
- 2 teaspoons red pepper flakes
- ½ cup chopped fresh cilantro
- Salt to taste
- A handful parsley leaves

1. Place a skillet over medium flame. Add oil and wait before it heats up. Add garlic and sauté for about a minute until light brown.
2. Stir in onions, tomatoes, jalapeño, parsley and red pepper flakes and cook for 4-5 minutes.
3. Stir the turkey and cook until the mixture is brown, breaking the turkey as it cooks.
4. Add cilantro, salt and pepper and stir.
Nutrition: Calories: 416 cal. – kcal: 1750 - Fat: 19 g - Protein: 45 g - Carbs:28 g - Sodium: 171.5 mg

268. Prawn & Coconut Curry

Preparation Time: 15 Minutes - Cooking Time: 40 -Minutes Servings: 1
- 400g (14oz) tinned chopped tomatoes
- 400g (14oz) large prawns (shrimps), shelled and raw
- 25g (1oz) fresh coriander (cilantro) chopped
- 3 red onions, finely chopped
- 3 cloves of garlic, crushed
- 2 bird's eye chillies
- ½ teaspoon ground coriander (cilantro)
- ½ teaspoon turmeric
- 400mls (14fl oz) coconut milk
- 1 tablespoons olive oil
- Juice of 1 lime

1. Place the onions, garlic, tomatoes, chilis, lime juice, turmeric, ground coriander (cilantro), chillies and half of the fresh coriander (cilantro) into a blender and blitz until you have a smooth curry paste. In a frying pan, heat the olive oil, add the paste and cook for 2 minutes. Stir in the coconut milk and warm it thoroughly. Add the prawns (shrimps) to the paste and cook them until they have turned pink and are completely cooked. Stir in the fresh coriander (cilantro). Serve with rice.

269. Orecchiette with Sausage and Chicory

Preparation time: 10 minutes - **Cooking time:** 20 – 25 minutes - **Servings:** 3
- ½ pound Orecchiette
- ½ pound sweet Italian sausage, discard casings
- ¼ teaspoon crushed red pepper
- Salt to taste

- 2 tablespoons grated pecorino + extra to garnish
- 2 tablespoons extra-virgin olive oil
- 1 clove garlic, peeled, thinly sliced
- ½ pound chicory or escarole, chopped
- ½ cup chicken stock
- A handful fresh mint leaves, chopped

1. Cook pasta following the package instructions, adding salt while cooking.
2. Place a large skillet over medium flame. Send the oil a tablespoon and let it heat up.
3. Once oil is heated, add sausage and cook until brown. Break it while it cooks.
4. With a slotted spoon, remove the sausage and put it on a plate.
5. Add a tablespoon of oil. Add garlic and red pepper when the oil is hot, and stir for a few seconds until you get a nice aroma.
6. Stir in chicory and salt and cook covered, until they turn limp. It should take a couple of minutes.
7. Uncover and continue cooking until tender.
8. Add pasta, sausage, cheese and stock and cook until the sauce is slightly thick. Add mint and stir.
Nutrition: 700 Calories 46 g Protein 25 g Carbohydrate 21 g Fat 14 g Saturated Fat 12 mg Cholesterol 93 mg Sodium

270. Lamb and Black Bean Chili

Preparation time: 10 minutes - **Cooking time:** 1 hour and 30 minutes - **Servings**: 4
- ¾ pound lean ground lamb
- 1 clove garlic, minced
- ½ cup dry red wine
- 1 teaspoon ground cumin
- Salt to taste
- Hot sauce to taste (optional)
- ½ cup chopped red onion
- 1 can (14.1 ounces) whole tomatoes, with its liquid, chopped
- ½ tablespoon chili powder
- 1 teaspoon dried oregano
- 1 ½ cans (15 ounces each) black beans, drained
- ½ teaspoon sugar
- Fresh cilantro sprigs (optional)

1. Place a Dutch oven over medium flame. Add lamb, onion and garlic and sauté until brown. Break it while you stir.

2. Use a slotted spoon to remove the mixture and place it on a board lined with paper towels. Discard the remaining fat in the pan. Wipe the pot clean.
3. Place the pot over medium flame. Add tomatoes, spices, oregano and salt and stir. Heat thoroughly.
4. Lower the heat and cook covered, for an hour. Add beans and hot sauce and stir.
5. Cover and simmer for about 30 minutes.
6. Sprinkle cilantro on top and serve.
Nutrition: Calories 270 Fat 13 g Cholesterol 15 mg Sodium 679 mg Potassium 696 mg Carbohydrates 15 g Fiber 6 g Sugar 4 g Protein 19 g

271. Tomato, Bacon and Arugula Quiche with Sweet Potato Crust

Preparation time: 15 minutes - **Cooking time:** 50 minutes - **Servings:** 8
- 4 cups shredded sweet potato or yam

- Salt to taste
- 1 red onion, chopped
- 2 large handfuls baby arugula
- 12 eggs
- 2 tablespoons olive oil
- 8 slices bacon, chopped
- 16 cherry tomatoes, quartered
- 6 cloves garlic, minced
- Pepper to taste
- 1 tablespoon butter or ghee

1. To make sweet potato crusts: You can grate the sweet potatoes on a box grater or in the food processor.
2. Squeeze excess moisture from the sweet potatoes.
3. Grease 2 pie pans (9 inches each) with some of the olive oil.
4. Add butter, pepper and salt into the bowl of sweet potatoes and mix well. Press the mixture onto the bottom and a little on the sides of the pie pan.
5. Bake the crusts in an oven preheated to 450° F, for around 20 minutes or until golden brown at the edges.
6. Remove the pie crusts from the oven.
7. Meanwhile, place a skillet over medium heat. Add bacon and cook until crisp. Place the bacon on a plate lined with paper towels with a slotted spoon. Discard the fat.
8. Add remaining oil into the skillet. Once oil is heated, add onions and sauté until it turns soft.
9. Stir in tomatoes and arugula and cook until the tomatoes are slightly soft.
10. Add in the garlic and cook for half a minute or so. Turn off the heat. Cool for a while.
11. Meanwhile, crack the eggs into a bowl. Add salt and pepper and whisk well.
12. Add the slightly cooled vegetables and bacon and stir.
13. Divide the egg mixture equally and pour over the baked sweet potato crust.
14. Place the crusts in the oven until the eggs are set, and bake.
15. Let it rest for 10 minutes.
16. Cut each into 4 wedges and serve.
Nutrition: Calories, 515 fat, 30g total carbohydrate, 6g fiber, 657mg sodium, 99g protein.

272. *Pomegranate Guacamole*

Preparation time: 10 Minutes - Cooking Time: 40 Minutes - Servings 4
- Flesh of 2 ripe avocados
- Seeds from 1 pomegranate
- 1 bird's-eye chili pepper, finely chopped ½ red onion, finely chopped
- Juice of 1 lime
- 151 calories per serving

1. Place the avocado, onion, chill and lime juice into a blender and process until smooth. Stir in the pomegranate seeds. Chill before serving. Serve as a dip for chop vegetables.

273. *Broccoli and Beef Stir-Fry*

Preparation Time: 5 minutes - **Cooking Time**: 18 minutes - **Servings**: 4
- 12 ounces frozen broccoli, thawed
- Sirloin beef, 8 ounces, sliced into thin strips
- 1 medium Roma tomato, chopped
- 1 teaspoon minced garlic
- 1 tablespoon cornstarch

- 2 tablespoons soy sauce, reduced-sodium
- ¼ cup chicken broth, low-sodium
- 2 tablespoons peanut oil
- 2 cups cooked brown rice

1. Take a frying pan, place it over medium heat, add oil and when hot, add garlic and cook for 1 minute until fragrant.
2. Add vegetable blend, cook for 5 minutes, then transfer vegetable blend to a plate and set aside until needed.
3. Add beef strips into the pan, and then cook for 7 minutes until cooked to the desired level.
4. Prepare the sauce by putting cornstarch in a bowl, and then whisking in soy sauce and broth until well combined.
5. Returned vegetables to the pan, add tomatoes, drizzle with sauce, stir well until coated, And cook until the sauce has thickened, for 2 minutes.
6. Serve with brown rice.
Nutrition: Calories: 373 kcal Total Fat: 17 g Saturated Fat: 0 g Cholesterol: 42 mg Sodium: 351 mg Total Carbs: 37 g Fiber: 5.1 g Sugar: 0 g Protein: 18 g

274. *Meatballs with Eggplant*

Preparation Time: 15 minutes - **Cooking Time:** 60 minutes - **Servings**: 6
- 1-pound ground beef
- ½ cup green bell pepper, chopped
- 2 medium eggplants, peeled and diced
- ½ teaspoon minced garlic
- 1 cup stewed tomatoes
- ½ cup white onion, diced
- 1/3 cup canola oil
- 1 teaspoon lemon and pepper seasoning, salt-free
- 1 teaspoon turmeric
- 1 teaspoon Mrs. Dash seasoning blend
- 2 cups of water

1. Take a large skillet pan, place it over medium heat, add oil in it and when hot, add garlic and green bell pepper and cook for 4 minutes until sauté.
2. Transfer the mixture of green pepper to a plate, set aside until required, then place the pieces of eggplant in the pan and cook until browned for 4 minutes per side and, when finished, transfer the eggplant to a plate and set aside until necessary.
3. Take a medium bowl, place beef in it, add onion, season with all the spices, Shape the mixture into 30 small meatballs and stir until well combined.
4. Place meatballs into the pan in a single layer and cook for 3 minutes, or until browned.
5. When done, place all the meatballs in the pan, add cooked bell pepper mixture in it along with eggplant, stir in water and tomatoes and simmer for 30 minutes at low heat setting until thoroughly cooked.
6. Serve straight away.
Nutrition: Calories: 265 kcal Total Fat: 18 g Saturated Fat: 0 g Cholesterol:47 mg Sodium: 153 mg Total Carbs: 12 g Fiber: 4.6 g Protein: 17 g

275. *Slow-Cooked Lemon Chicken*

Preparation Time: 20 minutes - **Cooking Time**: 7 hours - **Servings**: 4
- 1 teaspoon dried oregano
- ¼ teaspoon ground black pepper
- 2 tablespoons butter, unsalted
- 1-pound chicken breast, boneless, skinless
- ¼ cup chicken broth, low sodium

- ¼ cup water
- 1 tablespoon lemon juice
- 2 cloves garlic, minced
- 1 teaspoon fresh basil, chopped

1. In a small bowl, combine the oregano and ground black pepper. Rub the chicken with the mixture.
2. In a medium-size skillet over medium heat, melt the butter. In the melted butter, brown the chicken and then move the chicken to the slow cooker.
3. In the skillet, placed the chicken broth, water, lemon juice and garlic. Bring it to a boil so the browned bits are loosened from the skillet. Pour the chicken over it.
4. Cover, set the slow cooker for 2½ hours on high or 5 hours on low.
5. Add basil and baste chicken. Cover, cook on high for an additional 15–30 minutes or until chicken is tender.
Nutrition: Calories: 197 kcal Total Fat: 9 g Saturated Fat: 5 g Cholesterol: 99mg Sodium: 57 mg Total Carbs: 1 g Fiber: 0.3 g Sugar: 0 g Protein: 26 g

276. Pork with Pak Choi

Preparation Time: 15 Minutes - Cooking Time: 10 Minutes - Servings: 4

- 100g of shiitake mushrooms, sliced
- 1 tablespoon of corn flour
- 200g pak choi or choi sum-cut into thin slices 125ml of chicken stock
- 1 tablespoon of tomato purée
- 1 teaspoon of brown sugar
- 1 clove garlic, peeled and crushed
- 1 shallot, peeled and sliced
- 100g of bean sprouts
- 1 tablespoon of water
- 400g of pork mince (10% fat)
- 1 thumb (5cm) fresh ginger -peeled and grated 400g of firm tofu, cut into large cubes
- 1 tablespoon of rice wine
- 1 tablespoon of soy sauce
- A large handful (20g) of parsley, chopped 1 tablespoon of rapeseed oil

1.   Place the tofu on kitchen paper, cover it with kitchen paper, and then set it aside.

2.   Mix the water and corn flour in a small bowl and remove the lumps.Add in rice wine, brown sugar, chicken stock,tomato puree, and soy sauce. Also, add in the crushed ginger and garlic them mix.

3.   Place a large frying pan or wok on high heat and add oil to it. Add the mushrooms and stir-fry for 2 to 3 minutes until cooked and glossy. Using a slotted spoon, remove the mushrooms from the pan and let them rest. Add tofu to the pan, fry it until it is brown on all sides, when finished and set aside, extract it with a slotted spoon.

4.   Add the pak choi to your pan or wok, and stir-fry for about 2 minutes and, then add the mince. Cook it until it's cooked and then add the sauce to it. Reduce the heat by a notch and allow 12 minutes for the sauce to bubble around the meat.

5.   Add the tofu, beansprouts, and mushrooms to the pan and warm them all through. Remove it from the heat andmix in parsley then serve right away.

277. Chicken stir-fry

- 150g (5oz) egg noodles
- 50g (2oz) cauliflower flore ts, roughly chopped 25g (1oz) kale, finely chopped 25g (1oz) mange tout
- 2 sticks of celery, finely chopped 2 chicken breasts
- 1 red pepper (bell pepper), chopped 1 clove of garlic
- 2 tablespoons soy sauce
- 100mls (3½ fl oz) chicken stock (broth) 1 tablespoon olive oil

Servings 2, 566 calories per serving

1.   As per the instructions, cook the noodles and set them aside to keep warm. Heat the oil in a wok or a frying pan and add the garlic and chicken. Add in the kale, celery, cauliflower, red pepper (bell pepper), mange tout and cook for 4 minutes. Pour in the chicken stock (broth) and soy sauce and cook for 3 minutes or until the chicken is thoroughly cooked. Stir in the cooked noodles and serve.

278. Tuna with lemon herb dressing

Preparation time: 5 Minutes - Cooking Time: 15 Minutes - Servings: 4

- 4 tuna steaks 1 tablespoon olive oil For the dressing:
- 25g (1oz) pitted green olives, chopped 2 tablespoons fresh parsley, chopped 1 tablespoon fresh basil, chopped 2 tablespoons olive oil Freshly squeezed juice of 1 lemon Servings 4 241 calories per serving

1.   In a griddle pan, heat a tablespoon of olive oil. Add the tuna steaks and cook on a high heat for 2-3 minutes on each side. Reduce the cooking time if you want them rare. Place the dressing ingredients into a bowl and mix them well. Serve the tuna steaks with a dollop of dressing over them. Serve alongside a leafy rocket salad.

279. Kale, apple & fennel soup

Preparation time: 5 Minutes - Cooking Time: 20 Minutes - Servings: 4

- 450g (1lb) kale, chopped
- 200g (7oz) fennel, chopped
- 2 apples, peeled, cored and chopped 2 tablespoons fresh parsley, chopped 1 tablespoon olive oil
- Sea salt
- Freshly ground black pepper

1. In a saucepan, heat the oil, add the kale and fennel and cook for 5 minutes until the fennel softens. Stir in the parsley and apples. Cover and bring to a boil with hot water, and simmer for 10 minutes. Use a hand blender or blitz for food processing until the soup is smooth. With salt and pepper, season.

280. Lentil soup

Preparation time: 5 Minutes - Cooking Time: 25 Minutes - Servings: 4

- 175g (6oz) red lentils
- 1 red onion, chopped

- 1 clove of garlic, chopped
- 2 sticks of celery, chopped
- 2 carrots, chopped
- ½ bird's-eye chilli
- 1 teaspoon ground cumin
- 1 teaspoon ground turmeric
- 1 teaspoon ground coriander (cilantro) 1200mls (2 pints) vegetable stock (broth) 2 tablespoons olive oil
- Sea salt
- Freshly ground black pepper

1.   In a saucepan, heat the oil and add the onion and cook for 5 minutes. Put the carrots, lentils, celery, chilli, cilantro, cumin, turmeric, and garlic in the mixture and cook for 5 minutes. Pour the stock (broth) in, bring it to a boil, reduce the heat and simmer for 45 minutes. Purée the soup until smooth, using a hand blender or food processor. With salt and pepper, season. Just serve.

281. Cauliflower & walnut soup

Preparation time: 5 Minutes - Cooking Time: 15 Minutes - Servings: 4

- 450g (1lb) cauliflower, chopped 8 w alnut halves, chopped
- 1 red onion, chopped
- 900mls (1½ pints) vegetable stock (broth) 100mls (3½ fl oz)
- double cream (heavy cream) ½ teaspoon turmeric
- 1 tablespoon olive oil

1.   Heat the oil in a saucepan, add the cauliflower and red onion, and then cook, stirring continuously, for 4 minutes. Pour (broth) into the stock, bring to a boil and cook for 15 minutes. Stir in the turmeric, double cream and walnuts. Process the soup until smooth and fluffy, using a food processor or hand blender. Serve in bowls with a sprinkling of sliced walnuts and top off.

282. Celery & blue cheese soup

Preparation time: 5 Minutes - Cooking Time: 25 Minutes - Servings: 4

- 125g (4oz) blue cheese
- 25g (1oz) butter
- 1 head of celery (approx 65 0g) 1 red onion, chopped
- 900mls (1½ pints) chicken stock (broth) 150mls (5fl oz) single cream

1.   In a saucepan, heat the butter, add the onion and celery, and then cook until the vegetables soften. Pour the stock in, bring it to a boil, then reduce the heat and simmer for 15 minutes. Pour in the milk until it has melted and stir in the cheese. Serve right away and eat.

283. Spicy squash soup

Preparation time: 5 Minutes - Cooking Time: 35 Minutes - Servings: 4

- 150g (5oz) kale
- 1 butternut squash, peeled, de-seeded and chopped 1 red onion, chopped
- 3 bird's-eye chillies, chopped 3 cloves of garlic
- 2 teaspoons turmeric
- 1 teaspoon ground ginger
- 600mls (1 pint) vegetable stock (broth) 2 tablespoons olive oil

1.   In a saucepan, heat the olive oil, add the chopped butternut squash and onion and cook until tender, for 6 minutes. Add kale, garlic, chilli, turmeric and ginger and cook, stirring constantly, for 2 minutes. Bring it to a boil in the vegetable stock (broth) and simmer for 20 minutes. Use a food processor or a hand blender to smoothly process it. Serve alone or with a cream or crème fraiche swirl.

284. French onion soup

Preparation time: 5 Minutes - Cooking Time: 25 Minutes - Servings: 4

- 750g (1¾ lbs) red onions, thinly sliced 50g (2oz) cheddar cheese, grated (shredded) 12g (½ oz) butter
- 2 teaspoons flour
- 2 slices wholemeal bread
- 900mls (1½ pints) beef stock (broth) 1 tablespoon olive oil

1.   Heat the butter and oil in a large pan. Attach the onions and cook gently for 25 minutes on a low heat, stirring occasionally. Attach the flour and whisk well. Pour in and keep stirring in the stock (broth). Boil, minimize heat and simmer for 30 minutes. Bring to a boil. Cut the slices of bread into triangles, sprinkle with cheese and place them under a hot grill (broiler) until the cheese has melted. Serve the soup into bowls and add 2 triangles of cheesy toast on top.

285. Cream of broccoli & kale soup

Preparation time: 5 Minutes - Cooking Time: 35 Minutes - Servings: 4

- 250g (9oz) broccoli
- 250g (9oz) kale
- 1 potato, peeled and chopped
- 1 red onion, chopped
- 600mls (1 pint) vegetable stock 300mls (½ pint) milk
- 1 tablespoon olive oil
- Sea salt
- Freshly ground black pepper

1.   In a saucepan, heat the olive oil, add the onion and cook for 5 minutes. Put the potato, kale and broccoli into the mixture and cook for 5 minutes. Pour the stock (broth) and milk in and boil for 20 minutes. Process the soup until smooth and fluffy, using a food processor or hand blender. With salt and pepper, season. Re-heat and serve if desired.

286. Sesame miso chicken

Preparation time: 5 Minutes - Cooking Time: 40 Minutes - Servings 3

- 1 skinless cod fillet
- ½ cup buckwheat
- ½ red onion, sliced
- 2 stalks celery, sliced
- 10 green beans
- 2 cups kale, roughly chopped
- 3 sprigs of parsley
- 1 garlic clove, finely chopped
- 1 pinch cayenne or ½ chilli
- 1 tsp. Finely chopped fresh ginger
- 1 tsp. Sesame seeds
- 2 teaspoons of miso
- 1 tbsp. Mirin/ rice wine vinegar
- 1 tbsp. Extra virgin olive oil
- 1 tbsp. Of soy sauce 1 tsp ground turmeric

1. Coat the cod with a mixture of the miso, mirin and 1 teaspoon of the oil and set aside for 30 minutes up to one hour in the refrigerator.

2. Heat the oven to 400 f, then bake the cod for 10 minutes.

3. Sautee the onion and stir-fry in the oil that remains along with the green beans, kale, celery, chili pepper, garlic, ginger. Sautee until the kale is wilted but the beans and celery are tender. Add dashes of water if needed to the pan as you go.

4. Cook the buckwheat for 3 minutes with the turmeric according to the product instructions. To stir-fry, add the sesame seeds, parsley and tamari and serve with the greens and fish.

287. Sirt Salmon Salad

Preparation time: 5 Minutes - Cooking Time: 30 Minutes - Servings 1

- 1 large Medjool date, pitted then chopped
- 50g of chicory leaves
- 50g of rocket
- 1 tablespoon of extra-virgin olive oil
- 10g of parsley, chopped
- 10g of celery leaves, chopped
- 40g of celery, sliced
- 15g of walnuts, chopped
- 1 tablespoon of capers
- 20g of red onions-sliced
- 80g of avocado-peeled, stoned, and sliced Juice of ¼ lemon
- 100g of smoked salmon slices alternatives: lentils, tinned tuna, or cooked chicken breast

1. On a large plate, place all the salad leaves, then mix the rest of the ingredients and spread evenly on top of the leaves.

288. Red Onion Dhal

Preparation Time: 45 Minutes - Serves 4

- 1 tsp extra virgin olive oil
- 1 tsp mustard seeds
- 40g red onion, finely chopped
- 1 garlic clove, finely chopped
- 1 tsp finely chopped fresh ginger
- 1 bird's eye chili, finely chopped
- 1 tsp mild curry powder
- 2 tsp ground turmeric
- 300ml vegetable stock
- 40g red lentils, rinsed
- 50g kale
- 50ml tinned coconut milk
- 50g buckwheat

1. In a moderately sized sauce pan, warm the olive oil over a medium heat. Using the mustard seeds to ossify and fry until they begin to crackle. Add the garlic, ginger, chili and onion frying for 10 minutes, or until the onion is tender.

2. Throw in 1 tsp turmeric and curry powder, and then stir. Cook until fragrant for a few minutes, then pour in the

3. stock and bring to the boil. Pour in the lentils and cook for 30 minutes.

4. Add the coconut milk and kale, cooking for another 5 minutes or so. As the dhal is brewing, rinse the buckwheat with water and cook it according to packet Directions . Drain and serve with the dhal.

289. Tofu & Shiitake mushroom soup

Preparation Time: 15 Minutes - Serves 4

- 10g dried wakame
- 1L vegetable stock
- 200g shiitake mushrooms, sliced
- 120g miso paste
- 1* 400g firm tofu, diced
- 2 green onion, trimmed and diagonally chopped
- 1 bird's eye chili, finely chopped

1. Soak the wakame in lukewarm water for 10-15 minutes before draining.

2. In a medium-sized saucepan add the vegetable stock and bring to the boil. Toss in the mushrooms and simmer for 23 minutes.

3. Mix miso paste with 3-4 tbsp of vegetable stock from the saucepan, until the miso is entirely dissolved. Pour the miso-stock back into the pan and add the tofu, wakame, green onions and chili, then serve immediately.

290. Chicken Soup

Preparation Time: 25 Minutes - Cooking Time: 60 Minutes - Servings: 4

- 1 teaspoon of smoked paprika
- 300ml passata
- Salt and freshly ground black pepper
- 1 teaspoon of dried mixed herbs
- 1 x 400g can of black beans, drained

- 2 cloves garlic, peeled and crushed
- 1 carrot, peeled and roughly chopped
- 1 liter of water
- 1 teaspoon of mild chili powder
- 1 red chili, deseeded then finely chopped ½ teaspoon of turmeric
- 30g (large handful) of flat leaf parsley, chopped 1 x 400g can chopped tomatoes
- 1 teaspoon of paprika
- ½ teaspoon of ground cumin
- 1 green pepper, deseeded and chopped
- 1 x 400g can kidney beans, drained
- 4 chicken drumsticks
- 2 shallots, peeled then roughly chopped

1. Take a large saucepan and add in the chicken drumsticks, carrot, and shallots. Pour in the water and let it simmer.

2. Enable 20 minutes to cook, then with a spoon (slotted) remove the chicken drumsticks and set aside to cool.

3. Add in the chopped tomatoes, garlic, passata, chili, and green pepper, and let it simmer again. Put in the driedherbs, paprika, turmeric, smoked paprika, chili powder, and cumin, then simmer again for 30 minutes.

4. Pull off the skin from the chicken then pinch as much chicken as possible from the bone. Shred the chicken meat,place it on the pan along with the kidney beans and black beans, and cook for five minutes.

5. Remove from the sun, add and mix in the parsley. Season with salt and pepper (to taste).

291. Chicken curry with potatoes and kale
Preparation time: 10 Minutes - Cooking Time: 20 Minutes - Servings: 4

- 600g chicken breast, cut into pieces
- 4 tablespoons of extra virgin olive oil
- 3 tablespoons turmeric
- 2 red onions, sliced
- 2 red chilies, finely chopped
- 3 cloves of garlic, finely chopped
- 1 tablespoon freshly chopped ginger
- 1 tablespoon curry powder
- 1 tin of small tomatoes (400ml)
- 500ml chicken broth
- 200ml coconut milk
- 2 pieces cardamom
- 1 cinnamon stick
- 600g potatoes mainly waxy)
- 10g parsley, chopped
- 175g kale, chopped
- 5g coriander, chopped

1. Marinate the chicken in a teaspoon of olive oil and a tablespoon of turmeric for about 30 minutes. Then fry in a high frying pan at high heat for about 4 minutes. Remove from the pan and set aside.

2. In a pan with chili, garlic, onion and onion, heat a tablespoon of oil. From ginger. Boil all over medium heat, add the curry powder and a tablespoon of turmeric and cook,

stirring occasionally, for another two minutes. Add tomatoes, cook for another two minutes until finally chicken stock, coconut milk, cardamom and cinnamon stick are added. Cook for about 45 to 60 minutes and add some broth if necessary.

3. In the meantime, preheat the oven to 425 °. Peel and chop the potatoes. Bring water to the boil, add the potatoes with turmeric and cook for 5 minutes. Then pour off the water and let it evaporate for about 10 minutes. Spread olive oil together with the potatoes on a baking tray and bake in the oven for 30 minutes.

4. When the potatoes and curry are almost ready, add the coriander, kale and chicken and cook for five minutes until the chicken is hot.

5. Add parsley to the potatoes and serve with the chicken curry.

292. Paleo Chocolate Wraps with Fruits
Preparation time: 25 minutes - Cooking time: 0 minutes - Servings: 2

- 4 pieces Egg
- 100 ml Almond milk
- 2 tablespoons Arrowroot powder
- 4 tablespoons Chestnut flour
- 1 tablespoon Olive oil (mild)
- 2 tablespoons Maple syrup
- 2 tablespoons Cocoa powder
- 1 tablespoon Coconut oil
- 1-piece Banana
- 2 pieces Kiwi (green)
- 2 pieces Mandarins

1. Mix all ingredients (except fruit and coconut oil) into an even dough.

2. Melt some coconut oil in a small pan and pour a quarter of the batter into it.

3. Bake it like a pancake baked on both sides.

4. Place the fruit in a wrap and serve it lukewarm.

5. A wonderfully sweet start to the day!

293. Sirt Energy Balls
Preparation Time: 10 Minutes - Cooking Time: 40 Minutes - Servings: 20 balls

- 1 mug of mixed nuts (with plenty of walnuts) 7 Medjool dates
- 1 tablespoon of coconut oil
- 2 tablespoons of cocoa powder Zest of 1 orange (optional)

1. Start by placing the nuts in a food processor and grind them until almost powdered (more or less depending on thepreferred texture of your energy balls).

2. Add the Medjool dates, coconut oil, cacao powder, and run the blender again until fully mixed. Place the blend ina

refrigerator for half an hour, and then shape them into balls. You can add in the zest of an orange as you blend.

294. Kale and Tofu Curry

Preparation Time: 15 Minutes - Cooking Time: 40 Minutes - Servings: 12

- 1 red chili, deseeded and thinly sliced
- 1 teaspoon of salt
- 1 liter of boiling water
- 1 large onion, chopped
- ½ teaspoon of ground turmeric
- 200g of firm tofu, chopped into cubes
- ¼ teaspoon of cayenne pepper
- 4 cloves of garlic, peeled then grated
- 200g of kale leaves, stalks removed and torn ½ teaspoon of ground cumin
- 250g of dried red lentils
- 1 large thumb fresh ginger (about 7cm peeled then grated)
- 1 teaspoon of paprika
- 2 tomatoes, roughly chopped
- Juice of 1 lime
- 1 tablespoon of rapeseed oil
- 50g frozen soya edamame beans

1. Place a pan over low heat and add oil to it. Add in the onions and cook for five minutes, then add in chili, garlic, and ginger and cook for two more minutes. Add the salt, cayenne, paprika, turmeric, and cumin. Stir through then add in the red lentils and stir again.

2. Pour in boiling water and simmer for 10 minutes.

3. Reduce the heat and let it cook for another 20 to 30 minutes until the curry has the consistency of thick porridge. Add the soya beans, tomatoes, and tofu and let it cook for 5 minutes. Add the kale leaves, lime juice, and let it cook until the kale is tender. Serve.

295. Bean Stew

Preparation Time: 25 Minutes - Cooking Time: 40 Minutes - Servings: 4

- 50g of kale, chopped roughly
- ½ bird's eye chili, chopped finely (optional) 40g of buckwheat 50g of red onion, chopped finely
- 1 garlic clove, chopped finely
- 1 tablespoon of roughly chopped parsley 200ml vegetable stock
- 1 teaspoon of Herbes de Provence
- 200g of tinned mixed beans
- 1 teaspoon of tomato purée
- 1 x 400g tin of chopped Italian tomatoes
- 30g celery, trimmed and chopped finely
- 1 tablespoon of extra-virgin olive oil
- 30g of carrot, peeled and chopped finely

1. Heat oil over medium-low heat in a medium-sized saucepan. Add in the onion, celery, chili, carrot, garlic and herbs (if using) until the onions are soft enough but not colored.

2. Add the stock, tomato purée, and tomatoes and bring to a boil.

3. Put in the beans and allow for 30 minutes simmering.

4. Add the kales and cook for 5-10 minutes or until the kale is tender, and then add in parsley.

5. As it cools, cook the buckwheat as per the Directions on the packet. Drain the buckwheat and serve with thecooked stew.

296. Sirt Salmon Salad

Preparation Time: 10 Minutes - Cooking Time: 10 Minutes - Servings: 1

- 1 large Medjool date, pitt ed then chopped
- 50g of chicory leaves
- 50g of rocket
- 1 tablespoon of extra-virgin olive oil
- 10g of parsley, chopped
- 10g of celery leaves, chopped
- 40g of celery, sliced
- 15g of walnuts, chopped
- 1 tablespoon of capers
- 20g of red onions-sliced
- 80g of avocado-peeled, stoned, and sliced Juice of ¼ lemon
- 100g of smoked salmon slices (alternatives: lentils, tinned tuna, or cooked chicken breast)

1. On a large plate, place all the salad leaves, then combine the remaining ingredients and spread evenly on top of the leaves.

297. Roasted vegetable salad

Preparation time: 5 Minutes - Cooking Time: 20 Minutes - Servings: 4-5

- 3 tomatoes, halved
- 1 zucchini, quartered
- 1 fennel bulb, thinly sliced
- 2 small eggplants, ends trimmed, quartered
- 1 large red pepper, halved, deseeded, cut into strips
- 2 medium onions, quartered
- 1 tsp oregano
- 2 tbsp extra virgin olive oil

For the dressing

- 2/3 cup yogurt
- 1 tbsp fresh lemon juice1 small garlic clove, chopped

1. Place the zucchini, eggplant, pepper, fennel, onions, tomatoes and olive oil on a lined baking sheet. Season with salt, pepper and oregano and cook in an oven at 500 degrees F until golden, about 20 minutes.

2. Whisk the yogurt, lemon juice and garlic in a bowl. Taste and season with salt and pepper. Divide the vegetables in 4-5 plates. Top with the yogurt mixture and serve.

298. Warm leek and sweet potato salad

Preparation time: 5 Minutes - Cooking Time: 30 Minutes - Servings: 4-5

- 1.5lb sweet potato, unpeeled, cut into 1-inch pieces
- 4 small leeks, trimmed and cut into 1-inch slices
- 5-6 white mushrooms, halved
- 1 cup baby arugula le aves
- 2 tbsp extra virgin olive oil

For the dressing

- ½ cup yogurt 1 tbsp dijon mustard

1. Preheat oven to 350 f. Line a baking tray with baking paper. Place the sweet potato, leeks and mushrooms on the baking tray. Drizzle and toss with olive oil to coat. Roast until golden or for 20 minutes.

2. In a small bowl or cup, combine your yogurt and mustard. Place vegetables, mushrooms and baby arugula in a salad bowl and toss to combine. Serve drizzled with the yogurt mixture.

299. Chickpeas, Onion, Tomato & Parsley Salad in a Jar

Preparation time: 5 Minutes - Cooking Time: 50 Minutes - Servings 2

- 1 cup cooked chickpeas
- 1/2 cup chopped tomatoes
- 1/2 of a small onion, chopped
- 1 tbsp. chia seeds
- 1 Tbsp. chopped parsley

Dressing:

- 1 tbsp. olive oil and 1 tbsp. of Chlorella. 1 tbsp. fresh lemon juice and pinch of sea salt

1. Put ingredients in this order: dressing, tomatoes, chickpeas, onions and parsley.

300. Kale & Feta Salad with Cranberry Dressing

Preparation time: 5 Minutes - Cooking Time: 30 Minutes - Servings 2

- 9oz kale, finely chopped
- 2oz walnuts, chopped
- 3oz feta cheese, crumbled
- 1 apple, peeled, cored and sliced
- 4 medjool dates, chopped

For the Dressing

- 3oz cranberries
- ½ red onion, chopped
- 3 tablespoons olive oil
- 3 tablespoons water
- 2 teaspoons honey
- 1 tablespoon red wine vinegar

- Sea salt

1. In a food processor, place the ingredients for the dressing and process until smooth. You can add a little extra water if appropriate, if it seems too thick. Place all the ingredients in the salad in a bowl. Pour the dressing on and toss the salad into the mixture until it is well covered.

Salad

301. Spring Strawberry Kale Salad

Preparation Time: 5 minutes - Cooking Time: 15-20 minutes - Servings: 4

- 3 cups baby kale, rinsed and dried
- 10 large strawberries, sliced
- ½ cup honey
- 1/3 cup white wine vinegar
- 1 cup extra virgin olive oil
- 1 tablespoon poppy seeds
- 2 tablespoons pine nuts, toasted
- Salt and pepper to taste

1. Blend the baby kale with the strawberries in a big tub.
2. To make the dressing: In a blender, add the honey, vinegar, and oil and blend until smooth.
3. Stir in the seeds of the poppy and season to taste
4. Pour over the kale and strawberries and toss to coat.
Nutrition: Calories: 220cal Carbohydrates: 21g Fat: 15g Protein: 5g

302. Blackberry Arugula Salad

Preparation Time: 5 minutes - Cooking Time: 10 minutes - Servings: 5

- 3 cups baby arugula, rinsed and dried
- 1-pint fresh blackberries
- ¾ cups of crumbled feta cheese
- 1-pint cherry tomatoes, halved
- 1 green onion, sliced
- ¼ cup walnuts, chopped (optional)

To Serve:

- Balsamic reduction, as required

1. In a large bowl, toss together baby arugula, blackberries, feta cheese, cherry tomatoes, green onion, and walnuts.
2. Drizzle balsamic reduction over plated salads
Nutrition: Calories: 270 Fat: 13g Saturated Fat: 2g Carbohydrates: 38g

303. Apple Walnut Spinach Salad

Preparation Time: 5 minutes - Cooking Time: 10 minutes - Servings: 4

- 3 cups baby spinach
- 1 medium apple, chopped
- ¼ Medjool dates, chopped
- ¼ cup walnuts, chopped
- 2 tablespoons extra virgin olive oil
- 1 tablespoon sugar
- 1 tablespoon apple cider vinegar
- ½ teaspoon curry powder
- ¼ teaspoon turmeric
- 1/8 teaspoon chili pepper flakes
- ¼ teaspoon salt

74

1. Combine the spinach, apple, dates, and the walnuts in a wide bowl.
2. To make the dressing: In a jar with a tight-fitting lid, combine the remaining ingredients; shake well.
3. Drizzle over salad and toss to coat.
Nutrition: Calories: 166.1 Fat: 11.9g Cholesterol: 5.0g Carbohydrates: 12.6g

304. Enhanced Waldorf salad
Preparation Time: 5 minutes - **Cooking Time**: 2 hours - **Servings:** 4
- 4 – 5 stalks celery, sliced
- 1 medium apple, chopped
- ¼ cup walnuts, chopped
- 1 small red onion, diced
- 1 head of red endive, chopped
- 2 teaspoons fresh parsley, finely diced
- 1 tablespoon capers, drained
- 2 teaspoons Lovage or celery leaves, finely diced

For the dressing:
- 1 tablespoon extra-virgin olive oil
- 1 teaspoon balsamic vinegar
- 1 teaspoon Dijon mustard
- Juice of half a lemon

1. Whisk the milk, vinegar, mustard, and lemon juice together to make the dressing.
2. To a medium, large-sized salad bowl, add the remaining salad ingredients and toss.
3. Drizzle over the salad with the sauce, blend and serve cold.
Nutrition: Calorie: 582Kcal Fat: 103g Fat: 22.2g Protein: 8.2g

305. Kale Salad with Pepper Jelly Dressing
Preparation Time: 5 minutes - **Cooking Time:** 20 minutes - **Servings:** 4
- 4 tablespoons mild pepper jelly
- 3 tablespoons olive oil
- ¼ teaspoon salt
- ½ teaspoon Dijon mustard
- 3 cups baby kale leaves
- ½ cup goat cheese, crumbled
- ¼ cup walnuts, chopped

1. To make the dressing: whisk the pepper jelly, olive oil, salt and mustard together in a small cup.
2. Heat in the microwave for 30 seconds. Let cool.
3. In a wide bowl, put the kale and toss with the dressing. Serve topped with goat cheese and sprinkle with walnuts.
Nutrition: Calories: 1506.3 Kcal Cholesterol: 25.3mg Carbohydrates: 96.3g

306. Hot Arugula and Artichoke Salad
Preparation Time: 5 minutes - **Cooking time**: 10 minutes - **Servings:** 2
- 1 tablespoon extra-virgin olive oil
- 2 cups baby arugula, washed and dried
- 1 red onion, thinly sliced
- 1 (3/4 cups) jar marinated artichoke hearts, quartered or chopped
- 1 cup feta cheese, crumbled

1. Preheat oven to 300 degrees F.

2. Drizzle olive oil on a rimmed baking sheet. Spread arugula in a thick layer covering the baking sheet.
3. Arrange onions and artichokes over the spinach and drizzle the marinade from the jar over the entire salad.
4. Sprinkle with the cheese and bake until the arugula is wilted but NOT dry, or about 10 minutes.
5. Serve warm.
Nutrition: Calories: 281Kcal Fat: 26.g Cholesterol: 126mg Protein: 7g

307. Spinach and Chicken Salad
Preparation Time: 5 minutes - **Cooking Time:** 30 minutes - **Servings:** 4
- 2 cups of rinsed and dried fresh spinach
- 4 cooked halves of skinless, boneless chicken breast, sliced
- 1 zucchini, cut lengthwise in half and sliced
- 1 bell pepper red, chopped
- ½ cup of olives in black
- ¼ cup capers, drained
- ½ cups fontina cheese, frozen and shredded

1. On four salad plates, placed equal amounts of spinach.
2. Over spinach, arrange chicken, zucchini, bell pepper, and black olives and capers and top with spinach.
3. Cheese.
Nutrition: Calories: 120 Fat: 4.9g Cholesterol: 15mg Carbohydrates: 13g

308. Warm Citrus Chicken Salad
Preparation Time: 10 minutes - **Cooking Time:** 20 minutes - **Servings:** 4
- 3 cups torn fresh kale
- 2 mandarin oranges, peeled and pulled into individual segments ½ cup mushrooms, sliced
- 1 small red onion, sliced
- ½ pound skinless, boneless chicken breast halves - cut into strips ¼ cup walnuts, chopped
- 2 tablespoons extra virgin olive oil
- 2 teaspoons cornstarch
- ½ teaspoon ground ginger
- ¼ cup pure orange juice, fresh squeezed is best ¼ cup red wine vinegar or apple cider vinegar

1. The place was torn kale, orange segments, mushrooms, and onion into a large bowl and toss to combine.
2. In a skillet, sauté chicken and walnuts in oil stirring frequently until chicken is no longer pink, a minimum of 10 minutes.
3. In a small bowl, whisk the cornstarch, ginger, orange juice, and vinegar until smooth.
4. Stir into the chicken mixture. Bring to a boil and simmer, continually stirring for 2 minutes or until thickened and bubbly.
5. Serve salads and pour chicken mixture over the top.
Nutrition: Calories: 237 Fat: 11.3g Carbohydrates: 9.8g Cholesterol:101.9mg

309. Summer Buckwheat Salad
Preparation Time: 15 minutes - **Cooking time**: 30 minutes - **Servings:** 4
- ½ cup buckwheat groats
- ¾ cup corn kernels
- 2 medium-sized carrots, diced
- 1 spring onion, diced

- ¼ cucumber, chopped
- 1 red onion, diced
- 10 radishes, chopped
- 3 cups cooked black beans

1. Using a fine-mesh sieve, rinse the buckwheat under running water
2. Bring to a boil in 1 cup of water, and then reduce to a simmer, covered, for 10 minutes
3. Drain well and chill in the fridge for at least 30 minutes
4. Combine cooled buckwheat and remaining ingredients in a large salad bowl
Nutrition: Calories: 128 Fat: 22g Protein: 4g

310. *Greek-Style Shrimp Salad on a Bed of Baby Kale*

Preparation Time: 15 minutes - **Cooking Time:** 30 minutes - **Servings**: 4
- 1-pound raw shrimp (26 to 30), peeled
- ¼ cup extra virgin olive oil plus more, as needed for grilling
- Salt and pepper to taste
- Sugar to taste
- 2 medium tomatoes, diced
- ½ cup feta cheese, crumbled
- ½ cup black olives, sliced
- 1 teaspoon dried oregano
- 4 teaspoons red wine vinegar
- 3 cups of baby kale

1. Preheat a gas grill or barbeque on high.
2. Thread onto metal skewers with shrimp (or bamboo ones that have been soaked in water for 15 minutes).
3. Brush on both sides with oil, and season with salt, pepper, and sugar to taste.
4. Grill shrimp until spotty brown and fully cooked, about 2 minutes on each side.
5. Meanwhile, mix the tomatoes in a medium-sized dish,cheese, olives, oregano, 2 tablespoons. 2 teaspoons of vinegar and olive oil.
6. When the shrimp is cooked, unthread it carefully and add to bowl. Lightly toss all the ingredients to coat. Set aside.
7. When ready to serve, drizzle remaining oil over kale in a large bowl, tossing to coat. Add remaining vinegar and toss again.
8. Divide kale among 4 large plates. Top each of the shrimp mixture with a slice.
Nutrition: Calories: 460 Carbohydrates: 13g Fat: 33g Protein: 30g

311. *Walnut Herb Pesto*

Preparation Time: 5 minutes - **Cooking Time:** 3 Minutes - **Servings:** 4-6
- 1 cup walnuts
- ¾ cup parsley, chopped
- ¾ cup Lovage, chopped
- ¾ cup basil, chopped
- ½ cup Parmesan, grated
- 3 cloves of garlic, chopped
- ½ teaspoon salt
- ½ cup extra virgin olive oil

1. Mix all ingredients except olive oil in a food processor and pump for a couple of seconds to combine. To get the mixture

well pureed, you might need to scrape down the sides a few times.
2. Drizzle in the olive oil while the system is running to integrate the oil-once the oil is added, do not over the operation, 30 seconds is enough.
3. Serve with crisped baguette slices or pasta **Nutrition:** Calories: 31 Fat: 3.1g Carbohydrates: 0.8g

312. *Creamy Lovage Dressing*

Preparation Time: 5 minutes - **Cooking Time:** 0 mins - **Servings**: 2-3
- 1 lemon, juiced
- 1 teaspoon garlic powder
- 1 teaspoon dried onion powder
- 1 teaspoon Dijon mustard
- 1 teaspoon Lovage
- ¼ cup walnuts, soaked
- 1 teaspoon date or maple syrup
- Salt and pepper to taste

1. Blend the soaked nuts with the date syrup to make walnut butter.
2. Place all ingredients in a small mixing bowl.
3. Whisk well to combine.
Nutrition: Calories: 90Kcal Carbohydrates: 6g Fat: 8g Protein:0

313. *Sesame Tofu Salad*

Preparation Time: 12 minutes - **Cooking Time:** 30 minutes - **Servings**: 2
- Cooked tofu – 0.625g (shredded)
- Cucumber – 1 (peel, halve lengthways, deseed with a teaspoon and slice)
- Sesame seeds - 1 tablespoon
- Baby kale - 0.4375 g (roughly chopped)
- Red onion – ½ (shredded finely)
- Pak choi – ½ cup (shredded finely)
- Large handful (20g) parsley, chopped

For the Dressing
- Soy sauce - 2 teaspoon
- Sesame oil - 1 teaspoon
- Extra virgin olive oil - 1 tablespoon
- Juice of 1 lime
- Honey or maple syrup- 1 teaspoon

1. Sesame seeds are toasted in a dry frying pan for approx. Two minutes, until perfumed and lightly browned. To cool, pass the seeds onto a plate.
2. Mix the lime juice, soy sauce, honey, sesame oil, and olive oil in a small bowl to get your dressing.
3. Place the Pak choi, parsley, red onion, kale, and cucumber in a large bowl. Mix. Add to the bowl of the dressing and mix again.
4. Share the salad into two plates, and then add the shredded tofu on top. Sprinkle over the sesame seeds before you serve.
Nutrition: Total Fat: 200 Carbohydrate: 8g Fat: 12g Protein: 20g

314. *Turmeric Extract Poultry & Kale Salad with Honey Lime Dressing*

Preparation Time: 10 minutes - **Cooking time:** 30 minutes - **Servings:** 2
For the chicken:
- 1 teaspoon coconut oil
- 1/2 tool brown onion, diced

- 250-300 g/ 9 oz. hens mince or diced up her thighs
- 1 large garlic clove, finely diced
- 1 tsp turmeric powder
- 1teaspoon lime passion
- Juice of 1/2 lime
- 1/2 tsp salt + pepper

For the salad:
- 6 broccoli stalks or broccoli florets
- 2 tablespoons pumpkin seeds (pepitas).
- 3 huge kale leaves, stems eliminated and chopped.
- 1/2 avocado, sliced.
- Handful of fresh coriander leaves, chopped.
- Handful of fresh parsley leaves, sliced.

For the clothing:
- 3 tablespoons lime juice.
- 1 small garlic clove, finely grated.
- 3 tbsps. Extra-virgin olive oil (I made use of 1 tbsp. avocado oil and * 2 tbsps. EVO).
- 1 tsp raw honey.
- 1/2 tsp wholegrain or Dijon mustard.
- 1/2 teaspoon sea salt and pepper.

1. Melt the ghee or coconut oil over medium to high heat in a small frying pan. Include the onion and sauté on medium heat for 4-5 mins, until golden. Include the hen dice as well as garlic and mix for 2-3 minutes over medium-high warm, breaking it apart.

2. Add the turmeric extract, lime enthusiasm, lime juice, salt, and pepper, and cook, frequently mixing, for a further 3-4 mins. Establish the cooked dice apart.

3. While the poultry is cooking, bring a small saucepan of water to steam. Add the broccolini and prepare for 2 mins. Wash under cold water as well as cut into 3-4 pieces each.

4. Include the pumpkin seeds to the frying pan from the poultry and toast over tool warmth for 2 mins, often mixing to avoid burning season with a little salt. Allot. Raw pumpkin seeds are too high to make use of.

5. The area sliced Kale in a salad bowl as well as pour over the clothing. Utilizing your hands, throw as well as massage the Kale with the dress. This will undoubtedly soften the Kale, kind of like what citrus juice does to fish or beef carpaccio-- it 'cooks' it slightly.

6. Finally toss via the prepared hen, broccolini, fresh, natural herbs, pumpkin seeds, and avocado pieces.

Nutrition: Calories: 368 Carbohydrate: 30.3g Protein 6.7g Fat: 27.6g

315. Buckwheat Pasta with Chicken Kale & Miso Dressing

Preparation Time:15 minutes - **Cooking time:** 15 minutes - **Servings**: 2

For the noodles:
- 2-3 handfuls of kale leaves (eliminated from the stem as well as approximately cut).
- 150 g/ 5 oz. 100% buckwheat noodles.
- 3-4 shiitake mushrooms cut.
- 1 tsp coconut oil or ghee.
- 1 brownish onion carefully diced.
- 1 medium free-range chicken breast cut or diced.
- 1 long red chili very finely sliced (seeds in or out depending upon how warm you like it).
- 2 big garlic cloves finely diced.
- 2-3 tablespoons Tamari sauce (gluten-free soy sauce).

For the miso dressing:

- 1 1/2 tbsp. fresh, natural miso.
- 1 tbsp. Tamari sauce.
- 1 tbsp. extra-virgin olive oil.
- 1 tbsp. lemon or lime juice.
- 1 teaspoon sesame oil (optional).

1. Bring a tool saucepan of water to steam. Include the Kale as well as cook for 1 min, up until a little wilted. Remove as well as reserve yet schedule the water and bring it back to the boil. Add the soba noodles and chef according to the bundle guidelines (typically about 5 mins). Rinse under cold water and allotted.

2. Then pan fry the mushrooms in coconut oil (concerning a tsp) for 2-3 minutes until gently browned on each side. Sprinkle with sea salt and allotted.

3. In the very same frypan, warmth a lot more coconut oil or ghee over medium-high warm. Sauté onion and chili for 2-3 mins and then add the poultry pieces. Cook 5 mins over medium warmth, stirring a couple of times, after that, Garlic, tamari sauce, and a small splash of water are applied. Cook for an additional 2-3 mins,, often mixing till hen is cooked via.

4. Lastly, include the kale and soba noodles and toss with the poultry to warm up.

5. Mix the dressing and drizzle over the noodles right at the end of cooking; this way, you will certainly maintain all those beneficial probiotics in the miso to life as well as energetic.

Nutrition: Calories: 260 Carbohydrate: 35.3g Protein 15g Cholesterol: 50g Fat: 27.6g

316. Sirtfood Lentil Super Salad

Preparation Time: 10 minutes - **Cooking time:** 0 minutes - **Servings**: 1
- 20 g red onion, sliced
- 1 tbsp. extra virgin olive oil
- 1 large Medjool date, chopped
- 1 tbsp. capers
- ¼ cup rocket
- 2 avocados, peeled, stoned and sliced
- 100 g lentils
- ¼ cup chicory leaves
- 2 tbsp. chopped walnuts
- 1 tbsp. fresh lemon juice
- ¼ cup chopped parsley
- ¼ cup chopped celery leaves

1. Arrange salad leaves in a large bowl or a plate; mix the remaining ingredients well and serve over the salad leaves.

Nutrition: Calories: 456 Carbs: 54 Protein: 27 Fat: 11

317. Sirty Fruit Salad

Preparation Time: 10 minutes - **Cooking time:** 0 minutes - **Servings**: 1
- 10 blueberries
- 10 red seedless grapes
- ½ cup brewed green tea
- 1 apple, cored, chopped
- 1 tsp. honey
- 1 orange, chopped
- 2 tbsp. fresh lemon juice

1. Add honey into a cup of green tea and stir until dissolved; add orange juice and set aside to cool.

2. Place the chopped orange in a bowl and add grapes, apple and blueberries; Pour over the tea and leave to steep before serving for at least 5 minutes.

Nutrition: Calories per serving: 362.47 kcal Carbs per serving: 25.39 g Fats per serving: 9.34 g Proteins per serving: 5.28 g Fiber per serving: 2.86 g Sodium per serving: 9.

318. Superfood Cleansing Salad with Citrus Dressing

Preparation Time: 15 minutes - **Cooking time:** 0 minutes - **Servings**: 4

- 2 cups red cabbage, chopped
- 2 cups kale, chopped
- 1 head cauliflower, roughly chopped
- 1 red onion
- 2 cups baby carrots
- 1/3 cup fresh cilantro, chopped
- 1/3 cup sunflower seeds
- 1/2 cup raisins
- 1/2 cup raw hemp hearts Citrus Dressing:
- 2 tablespoons fresh lime juice
- 2 tablespoons fresh lemon juice
- 1/3 cup apple cider vinegar
- 1/2 avocado
- 2 cloves garlic
- 1/2 tablespoon fresh cilantro
- 1/2 tablespoon minced ginger
- 1/2 tablespoon raw honey
- 1/2 teaspoon sea salt
- 1/4 teaspoon pepper

1. Combine cabbage, kale, cauliflower, onion, carrots and cilantro in a food processor; shred.
2. Transfer the shredded veggies to a large bowl and fold in sunflower seeds, hemp hearts and raisins.
3. In a blender, mix all of the dressing ingredients and blend until very smooth.
4. Serve the salad in salad bowls drizzled with the citrus dressing. Enjoy!

Nutrition: Calories 91 kcal Fat 8.3 g Cholesterol 0 mg Carbohydrate 12.5 g Fat 0.5 g Protein 4. 4 g Sodium 810 mg

319. Sweet & Sour Bean Curry Salad

Preparation Time: 15 minutes - **Cooking time:** 40 minutes - **Servings**: 4

- ½ cup garbanzo beans, rinsed, drained
- 1 teaspoon extra virgin olive oil
- 1/8 teaspoon sea salt
- 2 teaspoons sunflower oil
- 2 teaspoons freshly squeezed lemon juice
- ½ teaspoon lemon zest
- ½ teaspoon raw honey
- A pinch of black pepper
- ¼ cup chopped bird eye's chili pepper
- 1 peeled mandarin orange, chopped
- ½ cup chopped purple cabbage
- ½ cup cooked quinoa
- 1 tablespoon toasted walnuts

1. On a baking sheet, spread the beans and bake at 450 °F for about 30 minutes or until lightly browned and slightly crunchy. Remove the beans from oven and let cool completely.

2. Toss together the baked beans, oil, and salt and return to oven for 10 more minutes or until crispy and browned. Remove from oven and let cool.
3. Whisk the sunflower oil, lemon juice, zest, sugar, sea salt and black pepper together in a bowl; set aside.
4. In a bowl, toss together the roasted beans with chopped mandarin orange, bird's eye chili pepper, cabbage and cooked quinoa; drizzle with the dressing and sprinkle with toasted walnuts to serve.

Nutrition: Calories: 534 calories Fat: 6 g Sodium: 693 mg Carbohydrates:89.7 g Fiber: 2.1 g Sugar: 53 g Protein: 20. 2 g

320. Strawberry & Cucumber Salad

Preparation Time: 10 minutes - **Cooking time:** 0 minutes - **Servings**: 1

- 8 strawberries, sliced
- 1 cucumber, sliced
- Pinch of sea salt
- Pinch of white pepper
- Stevia

Dressing:
- 4 tablespoons fresh lemon juice
- 1 tablespoon extra-virgin olive oil
- 1 tablespoon apple cider vinegar
- ½ cup chopped strawberries
- Pinch of salt
- Pinch of pepper

1. Mix the salad ingredients in a big tub, in a blender, blend together dressing ingredients until smooth and pour over the salad. Toss to coat well and serve.

Nutrition: Calories - 8 (700 kg.), P - 0.24 g, F - 0.02 g, C - 0. 58 g, Sodium - 0.30 e%, Omega-6 - 0.02 g, Omega-3 - 0.05 g.

321. Sweet Kale & Cranberry Salad

Preparation Time: 20 minutes - **Cooking time:** 0 minutes - **Servings**: 6

- 2 large peeled sweet potatoes, cubed
- 2 bunches kale, chopped into small pieces
- 1 tablespoon fresh lemon juice
- 3 tablespoons extra-virgin olive oil
- 1/4 cup Sunflower seeds
- ½ cup toasted walnuts, chopped
- 1/2 cup dried cranberries
- 1 teaspoon Dijon mustard
- A pinch of sea salt
- A pinch of freshly ground pepper

1. In a medium saucepan, put the potatoes and cover with water; stir in a pinch of salt and bring to a gentle boil. Simmer and simmer for about 15 minutes or until the potatoes are soft; drain and cool for about 15 minutes.
2. Whisk the mustard, lemon juice and extra virgin olive oil together in a large cup.
3. Add the sweet potatoes along with all the remaining ingredients; toss to mix well and serve.

Nutrition: 25 grams of sugar, 225 calories

322. Super Raw Power Salad

Preparation Time: 10 minutes - **Cooking time:** 0 minutes - **Servings**: 8

For the Dressing:
- ¼ cup white apple cider vinegar
- ¾ cup extra virgin olive oil

- 1 tablespoon raw honey
- 1/8 teaspoon garlic powder
- 1/8 teaspoon sea salt
- 2 apples, finely chopped
- ½ cup bean sprouts
- ½ cup frozen edamame, thawed
- ¾ cup dried berries
- 1½ cups chopped purple cabbage
- 4 cups finely chopped kale
- ½ cup raw sunflower seeds
- Pinch of sea salt
- Pinch of pepper

1. In a sealable jar, mix all dressing ingredients and shake until well blended.
2. In a large bowl, mix all salad ingredients; pour about ¼ cup of the dressing over the salad and toss to coat well. Season with salt and pepper and serve.
Nutrition: 426 calories, 6g protein, 94g carbs, 18g fat, 171mg sodium

323. *Apple, Carrot, Cucumber & Mixed Greens Salad w/ Raspberry Vinaigrette*

Preparation Time: 10 minutes - **Cooking time:** 0 minutes - **Servings**: 1
- 1 cup microgreens
- 1/2-pound mixed greens
- 1/2 tart apple, chopped
- 1/2 small cucumber, thinly sliced
- 3 carrots, sliced
- 1 tablespoon sherry vinegar
- 2 tablespoons extra virgin olive oil
- 1 tablespoons mustard
- Handful of blueberries
- Pinch of sea salt
- Pinch of pepper
- 1 hardboiled egg, chopped

1. In a large bowl, combine microgreens, mixed greens, apple, cucumber, and carrots.
2. Combine sherry vinegar, olive oil, mustard, blueberries, salt and pepper in a sealable jar; shake vigorously to combine well and pour over the salad. Serve on plates topped with chopped hardboiled egg.
Nutrition: Calories: 177 Total fat: 22 g Saturated fat: 3.9 g Carbohydrates:14.3 g Sugar: 11.2 g Fiber: 5.2 g Protein: 3.2 g Sodium: 123 mg

324. *Sirtfood Salad with Citrus Dressing*

Preparation Time: 25 minutes - **Cooking time:** 0 minutes - **Servings**: 6
For salad
- 2 cup red cabbage, finely sliced
- 2 cup kale, finely sliced
- 1 cup parsley, chopped
- 1 bird eye's chili, diced
- 1 cup radish, sliced in matchsticks
- 2 cup broccoli, chopped in ¼-inch pieces
- 1 cup carrot, sliced in matchsticks
- 1 cup raw walnuts, chopped
- 2 avocados, peeled and diced
- 2 tablespoons sesame seeds
- freshly ground black pepper to taste
- ½ cup fresh lemon juice

- ½ cup fresh orange juice
- ½ cup extra-virgin olive oil
- 1 teaspoon minced ginger
- 1 tablespoon raw honey
- Pinch of cayenne
- ¼ teaspoon sea salt

1. Process dressing ingredients until very smooth.
2. Combine salad ingredients in a salad bowl; pour the dressing over the salad and toss to combine well. Enjoy!
Nutrition: carb: 37.9g, fat: 14.8g, protein: 57.

325. *Kale Avocado Salad with Orange*

Preparation Time: 10 minutes - **Cooking time:** 0 minutes - **Servings**: 2
Salad
- 2-3 handfuls kale, rinsed and chopped
- ½ cup green peas
- ½ avocado, sliced
- ½ cucumber, sliced
- 1 orange, sliced
- 2 tablespoons chopped toasted walnut
- 2 tablespoons hemp seeds, shelled Vinaigrette
- 2 tablespoons extra virgin olive oil
- 3 tablespoons lemon juice
- Pinch garlic powder
- Sea salt
- Black pepper

1. In a saucepan, place the chopped kale. In a small bowl, mix extra virgin olive oil, lemon juice, garlic powder, sea salt and pepper; rub the lemon vinaigrette with your hands into the kale for approximately 2 minutes or until the kale begins to soften.
2. Divide the between two serving plates and add peas, avocado, cucumber, and orange slices.
3. Top with almond slices and hemp seeds; drizzle with lemon juice and sprinkle with cracked pepper. Enjoy!
Nutrition: Calories: 80g Total fat: 6.6g Protein: 1.6g Carbohydrate: 1. 5g
Sugar: 0.3g Sodium: 0. 5g

326. *Caesar Dressing*

Preparation Time: 10 minutes - **Cooking Time:** 5 minutes - **Servings**: 1 cup
- 250 ml Olive oil
- 2 tablespoons Lemon juice
- 4 pieces Anchovy fillet
- 2 tablespoon Mustard yellow
- 1 clove Garlic
- ½ teaspoon Salt
- ½ teaspoon Black pepper

1. Remove the garlic peel and finely chop it.
2. Put all ingredients in a blender and puree evenly.
3. It is possible to keep this dressing for about 3 days in the fridge.
Nutrition: Calories: 71 Cal Fat: 2.78 g Carbs: 6.76 g Protein: 6.38 g Fiber: 2.1 g

327.   *Basil Dressing*

Preparation Time: 10 minutes - **Cooking Time:** 5 minutes - **Servings**: 1 cup
- 100 g fresh basil
- 1 pc Shallots
- 1 clove Garlic

- 125 ml Olive oil (mild)
- 2 tbsp White wine vinegar

1. Finely chop the shallot and garlic.
2. Put the shallot, garlic, basil, olive oil and vinegar in a blender.
3. Mix it into an even mix.
4. Season the dressing and season with salt and pepper.
5. Place the dressing in a clean glass and store in the refrigerator. It stays fresh and tasty for at least 3 days.
Nutrition: Calories: 33 Cal Fat: 0.66 g Carbs: 3.72 g Protein: 3.35 g Fiber: 1.7 g

328. Strawberry Sauce

Preparation Time: 15 minutes - **Cooking Time:** 15 minutes - **Servings:** 1 cup
- 225 g Strawberries
- 3 tablespoons Coconut blossom sugar
- 4 tablespoons Honey
- 125 ml Water
- 2 teaspoon Arrowroot powder

1. Roughly chop strawberries.
2. Put the strawberries in a pan with coconut blossom sugar and honey. Place the pan on medium heat.
3. In the meantime, mix the arrow roots with a whisk in the water. Add this mixture to the strawberries.
4. Heat the strawberries until they start to bubble and start to thicken. (Not cook!)
5. Your strawberry sauce is ready after about 15 minutes. Store the sauce in a clean glass refrigerator.
Nutrition: Calories: 238 Cal Fat: 3.91 g Carbs: 105.68 g Protein: 2.81 g Fiber: 5.4 g

329. Fresh Chicory Salad

Preparation Time: 15 minutes - **Cooking Time:** 5 minutes - **Servings:** 2 – 3
- 1 piece Orange
- 1 piece Tomato
- ¼ pieces Cucumber
- 1/4 pieces Red onion

1. Cut off the hard stem of the chicory and remove the leaves.
2. Peel the orange and cut the pulp into wedges.
3. Break the cucumbers and tomatoes into small bits.
4. Cut the red onion into thin half rings.
5. Place the chicory boats on a plate, spread the orange wedges, tomato, cucumber and red onion over the boats.
6. Sprinkle some olive oil and fresh lemon juice on the dish.
Nutrition: Calories: 73 Cal Fat: 0.49 g Carbs: 15.73 g Protein: 2.68 g Fiber: 3.5 g

330. Grilled Vegetables And Tomatoes

Preparation Time: 10 minutes - **Cooking Time:** 10 minutes - **Servings:** 2 – 3
- 1 piece Zucchini
- 1 piece Eggplant
- 3 pieces Tomatoes
- 1 piece Cucumber

Dressing:
- 4 tablespoons Olive oil
- 110 ml Orange juice (fresh)
- 1 tablespoon Apple cider vinegar
- 1 hand fresh basil

1. Cut all of the vegetables into equally thick slices (about half a centimeter).
2. Heat the grill pan and fry the zucchini and eggplant.
3. While the zucchini and eggplant are fried, season with salt and pepper.
4. Remove the basil leaves from the branches.
5. Spread the vegetables alternately on a plate.
6. Add a leaf of basil every now and then.
7. Mix the ingredients for the dressing and serve the dressing separately on the side.
Nutrition: Calories: 168 Cal Fat: 55.53 g Carbs: 40.39 g Protein: 7.7 g Fiber: 18.7 g

331. Steak Salad

Preparation Time: 10 minutes - **Cooking Time:** 10 minutes - **Servings:** 2 – 3
- 2 pieces Beef steak
- 2 cloves Garlic
- 1 piece Red onion
- 2 pieces Egg
- 1 hand Cherry tomatoes
- 2 hands Lettuce
- 1 piece Avocado
- ½ pieces Cucumber
- 1 pinch Season white Salt
- 1 pinch Black pepper

1. Place the steaks in a flat bowl.
2. Pour the olive oil over the steaks and press the garlic over it. Turn the steaks a few times so that they are covered with oil and garlic.
3. Cover the meat and allow it to marinate for at least 1 hour.
4. Boil eggs.
5. Heat a grill pan and fry the steaks medium.
6. Take the steaks out of the pan, wrap them in aluminum foil and let them rest for 5 to 10 minutes.
7. Spread the lettuce on the plates.
8. Cut the steaks into slices and place them in the middle of the salad.
9. Cut the eggs into wedges, the cucumber into half-moons, the red onion into thin half-rings, cherry tomatoes into halves and slices of avocado.
10. Spread this around the steaks.
11. Sprinkle over the olive oil and white wine vinegar and season with a little salt and pepper.
Nutrition: Calories: 131 Cal Fat: 74.9 g Carbs: 37.09 g Protein: 23 g Fiber: 17 g

332. Zucchini Salad With Lemon Chicken

Preparation Time: 1 hour 10 minutes - **Cooking Time:** 25 minutes - **Servings:** 2 – 3
- 1 piece Zucchini
- 1 piece yellow zucchini
- 1 hand Cherry tomatoes
- 2 pieces Chicken breast
- 1 piece Lemon
- 2 tablespoons Olive oil

1. Utilize a meat mallet or a heavy pan to make the chicken fillets as thin as possible.
2. Put the fillets in a bowl.
3. Over the chicken, squeeze the lemon and apply the olive oil. Cover it and leave for at least 1 hour to marinate.
4. Heat a pan over medium-high heat and fry the chicken until cooked through and browned.
5. Season with salt and pepper.

6. Make zucchini from the zucchini and put in a bowl.

7. Quarter the tomatoes and stir in the zucchini.

8. Slice the chicken fillets diagonally and place them on the salad.

9. Drizzle a little olive oil with the salad and season with salt and pepper.

Nutrition: Calories: 125 Cal Fat: 80.83 g Carbs: 4.97 g Protein: 121.48 g Fiber: 0.4 g

333. *Fresh Salad With Orange Dressing*

Preparation Time: 10 minutes - **Cooking Time:** 5 minutes - **Servings:** 2 – 3

- 1 / 2 fruit Salad
- 1 piece yellow bell pepper
- 1 piece Red pepper
- 100 g Carrot (grated)
- 1 hand Almonds

Dressing:

- 4 tablespoon Olive oil
- 110 ml Orange juice (fresh)
- 1 tablespoon Apple cider vinegar

1. Clean the peppers and cut them into long thin strips.

2. Tear off the lettuce leaves and cut them into smaller pieces.

3. Mix the salad with the peppers and the carrots processed with the Julienne peeler in a bowl.

4. Chop the almonds roughly and scatter over the salad.

5. In a tub, combine all the ingredients for the dressing. Just prior to eating, pour the dressing over the salad.

Nutrition: Calories: 158 Cal Fat: 55.07 g Carbs: 16.84 g Protein: 2.76 g Fiber: 4.5 g

334. *Tomato And Avocado Salad*

Preparation Time: 10 minutes - **Cooking Time:** 5 minutes - **Servings:** 2 – 3

- 1 piece Tomato
- 1 hand Cherry tomatoes
- ½ pieces Red onion
- 1 piece Avocado
- Taste fresh oregano
- 1 1 / 2 EL Olive oil
- 1 teaspoon White wine vinegar
- 1 pinch Celtic sea salt

1. Cut the tomato into thick slices.

2. Cut half of the cherry tomatoes into slices and the other half in half.

3. Cut the red onion into super thin half rings. (or use a mandolin for this)

4. Cut the avocado into 6 parts.

5. Spread the tomatoes on a plate, place the avocado on top and sprinkle the red onion over them.

6. Sprinkle fresh oregano on the salad as desired.

7. Drizzle olive oil and vinegar on the salad with a pinch of salt.

Nutrition: Calories: 138 Cal Fat: 29.65 g Carbs: 29.86 g Protein: 5.6 g Fiber: 15.8 g

335. *Arugula With Fruits And Nuts*

Preparation Time: 10 minutes - **Cooking Time:** 5 minutes - **Servings:** 2 – 3

- 75 g Arugula
- 2 pieces Peach
- ½ pieces Red onion
- 1 hand Blueberries
- Pecans 1 hand

Dressing:

- ½ pieces Peach
- 65 ml Olive oil
- 2 tablespoon White wine vinegar
- 1 sprig fresh basil
- 1 pinch Salt
- 1 pinch Black pepper

1. Halve the 2 peaches and remove the core.

2. Cut the pulp into pieces.

3. Heat a grill pan and grill the peaches briefly on both sides.

4. Cut the red onion into thin half rings.

5. Roughly chop the pecans.

6. Heat a pan and roast the pecans in it until they are fragrant.

7. Place the arugula on a plate and spread it over the peaches, red onions, blueberries and roasted pecans.

8. Place all the dressing ingredients in a blender or food processor and mix with a smooth dressing.

9. Drizzle the dressing over the salad.

Nutrition: Calories: 68 Cal Fat: 0.61 g Carbs: 13.09 g Protein: 3.16 g Fiber: 3.1 g

336. *Spinach Salad With Green Asparagus And Salmon*

Preparation Time: 10 minutes - **Cooking Time:** 5 minutes - **Servings:** 2 – 3

- 2 hands Spinach
- 2 pieces Egg
- 120 g smoked salmon
- 100 g Asparagus tips
- 150 g Cherry tomatoes
- Lemon ½ pieces
- 1 teaspoon Olive oil

1. Make the eggs the way they please you.

2. Heat a pan with a little oil and fry the asparagus tips al dente.

3. Halve cherry tomatoes.

4. Place the spinach on a plate and spread the asparagus tips, cherry tomatoes and smoked salmon on top.

5. Scare, peel and halve the eggs. Add them to the salad.

6. Squeeze the lemon over the lettuce and drizzle some olive oil over it.

7. Season the salad with a little salt and pepper.

Nutrition: Calories: 208 Cal Fat: 32.92 g Carbs: 33.24 g Protein: 46.65 g Fiber: 5.4 g

337. *Brunoise Salad*

Preparation Time: 10 minutes - **Cooking Time:** 5 minutes - **Servings:** 1

- 1 piece Meat tomato
- ½ pieces Zucchini
- ½ pieces Red bell pepper
- ½ pieces yellow bell pepper
- ½ pieces Red onion
- 3 sprigs fresh parsley
- ½ pieces Lemon
- 2 tablespoons Olive oil

1. Finely dice the tomatoes, zucchini, peppers and red onions to get a brunoise.

2. Mix all the cubes in a bowl.

3. Chop parsley and mix in the salad.

4. Over the salad, squeeze the lemon and apply the olive oil.

5. Season with salt and pepper.

Nutrition: Calories: 268 Cal Fat: 28.06 g Carbs: 28.39 g Protein: 5.64 g Fiber: 5.4 g

338. Broccoli Salad

Preparation Time: 10 minutes - **Cooking Time:** 5 minutes - **Servings:** 1

- 1 piece Broccoli
- ½ pieces Red onion
- 100 g Carrot (grated)
- 1 hand Red grapes

Dressing:

- 2 ½ tablespoon Coconut yogurt
- 1 tablespoon Water
- 1 teaspoon Mustard yellow
- 1 pinch Salt

1. Slice the broccoli into small florets and cook al dente for 5 minutes.

2. Cut the red onion into thin half rings.

3. Halve the grapes.

4. Mix coconut yogurt, water and mustard with a pinch of salt to make an even dressing.

5. Drain the broccoli and rinse with ice-cold water to stop the cooking process.

6. Mix the broccoli with the carrot, onion and red grapes in a bowl.

7. Serve the dressing separately on the side.

Nutrition: Calories: 91 Cal Fat: 0.52 g Carbs: 20.79 g Protein: 2.41 g Fiber: 5.4 g

339. Kale & Feta Salad

Preparation Time: 10 minutes - **Cooking Time:** 0 minute - **Servings:** 1

- 250g kale, finely chopped
- 50g walnuts, chopped
- 75g feta cheese, broken
- 1 apple, peeled, cored & diced
- 4 medjool dates, chopped
- 75g cranberries
- ½ red onion, chopped
- 3 tbsp. olive oil
- 3 tbsp. water
- 2 tsp honey, 1 tbsp. red wine vinegar
- A pinch of salt

1. In a bowl, throw together the kale, walnuts, feta cheese, apple, and dates, and then stir.

2. In a food processor, add cranberries, red onion, olive oil, water, honey, red wine vinegar, and a pinch of salt. Process until smooth and fluid, adding water if necessary. Pour the cranberry dressing over the salad and serve.

Nutrition: Calories: 186 Fiber: 2.5 g

340. Crowning Celebration Chicken Salad

Preparation Time: 5 minutes - **Cooking Time:** 10 minutes - **Servings:** 1

- 75 g Natural yogurt
- Juice of 1/4 of a lemon
- 1 tsp Coriander, cleaved
- 1 tsp Ground turmeric
- 1/2 tsp Mild curry powder
- 100 g Cooked chicken bosom, cut into scaled down pieces

- 6 Walnut parts, finely shredded
- 1 Medjool date, finely shredded
- 20 g Red onion, diced
- 1 Bird's eye bean stew
- 40 g Rocket, to serve

1. Blend the yogurt, lemon juice, coriander and flavors together in a bowl.

2. Attach all of the remaining ingredients and serve on the rocket bed.

Nutrition: Calories 314 Fat: 13 g Carbohydrates: 28 g Protein: 2 g Fiber:1 g

341. Sirt Super Salad

Preparation Time: 15 Minutes - **Cooking Time:** 15 Minutes - **Servings:** 1

- 1 ¾ ounces (50g) arugula
- 1 ¾ ounces (50g) endive leaves
- 3 ½ ounces (100g) smoked salmon cuts
- ½ cup (80g) avocado, stripped, stoned, and cut 1/2 cup (50g) celery including leaves, cut 1/8 cup (20g) red onion, cut 1/8 cups (15g) pecans, shredded
- 1 tablespoon escapades
- 1 enormous Medjool date, hollowed and shredded
- 1 tablespoon additional virgin olive oil
- juice of ¼ lemon
- ¼ cup (10g) parsley, shredded

1. Spot, the serving of mixed greens, leaves on a plate or in an enormous bowl.

2. Combine and serve over the leaves with all the rest of the ingredients.

Nutrition: Calories 236 Fat: 13 g Carbohydrates: 28 g Protein: 2 g

342. Walnuts Avocado Salad

Preparation Time: 8 minutes - **Cooking Time:** 0 minutes - **Servings:** 1

- ¼ cup of chopped parsley
- ¼ lemon juice
- 1 tbsp. of extra virgin olive oil
- 1 large Medjool date, pitted and chopped
- 1 tbsp. of capers
- 1/8 cups of chopped walnuts
- 1/8 cup of sliced red onion
- ½ cup of celery including leaves, sliced
- ½ cup of avocado, peeled, stoned, and sliced 100 grams of smoked salmon slices (3 ½ oz.) 50 grams of endive leaves (1 ¾ oz.)
- 50 grams of arugula (1 ¾ oz.)

1. Place the endive leaves, parsley, celery leaves and arugula in a large bowl or plate.

2. Mix together the remaining ingredients and serve over of the leaves.

Nutrition: Calories 89 Sugar 2 Carbohydrate 33 Vitamin K and C

343. Poached Pear Salad with Dijon Vinegar Dressing

Preparation Time: 15 minutes - **Cooking Time:** 0 minutes - **Servings:** 1

For The Dressing

- 75 ml olive oil
- 75 ml walnut oil

- 1 tbsp. of red wine vinegar
- 1 tbsp. of Dijon mustard
- Freshly ground Pepper to taste
- Salt to taste

For The Salad
- 200 grams of Gorgonzola cheese, slice finely Few rocket leaves
- 100 grams of Walnuts
- 2 Ripe pears (peeled and core) cut into quarters
- 2 Bay leaves
- Small bunch of thyme
- 40 grams of caster sugar
- 180 ml of red wine

1. Boil the wine in a saucepan. Along with the bay leaves, sugar and thyme. Simmer over medium-low heat.
2. Add the pear into the simmering liquid and poach for 10 minutes. Remove from the heat of the pan and set aside in poaching fluid to cool pears.
3. Mix the mustard, salt, vinegar, and pepper together in a bowl until well whisked; steam in the oil slowly and whisk as you apply.
4. Arrange salad ingredients on a serving plate and drizzle with the dressing.
Nutrition: Calories 88 Sugar 4 Carbohydrate 24

344. Steak Arugula Strawberry Salad
Preparation Time: 10 minutes - **Cooking Time:** 15 minutes - **Servings:** 4
Steak:
- 1/2 tbsp. extra virgin olive oil
- Montreal steak seasoning
- 2 Beef tenderloin steaks

Salad:
- 1/8 cup of slivered walnuts
- 1/4 cup of crumbled feta cheese
- 1/2 cup of sliced strawberries
- 1/2 cup blueberries
- 1/2 cup of raspberries
- 3 cups of arugula
- Balsamic Vinaigrette
- Salt and pepper
- 1/4 tsp of Dijon mustard
- 1 1/2 tsp of sugar
- 1/8 cup of olive oil
- 1/8 cup of balsamic vinegar

Directions:
1. Steak:
2. Run the Montreal steak seasoning all over the steak and let sit for 5-10 minutes.
3. Heat oil over medium high heat in a cast-iron skillet. Once it's simmering, add in the steak and cook about 5-7 minutes; flip and cook the other side for 3-4 minutes or until its cooked the way you like your meet.
4. Set steak aside in a plate and let cool for 5 minutes before slicing into strips.
5. Salad:
6. Combine together the salad ingredients in a large bowl.
7. In a small shaker, add together the all vinaigrette ingredients and shake until well mixed. Pour the dressing over the lettuce and toss to cover evenly.
8. To Serve
9. Divide the salad into 2 bowls, then cover it with the steak.
10. Notes:

11. You can keep the dressing for up to one week in the fridge.
Nutrition: kcal: 506 Net carbs: 17g Fat: 37g Fiber: 5g Protein: 23 g

345. Super Fruit Salad
Preparation Time: 10 minutes - **Cooking Time:** 0 minutes - **Servings:** 1
- 10 blueberries
- 10 red seedless grapes
- 1 apple, cored and chopped roughly
- 1 orange, halved
- 1 tsp of honey
- ½ cup of freshly made matcha green tea

1. Combine 1/2 cup green tea with the honey and stir until dissolved, Squeeze in half of the orange into the green tea mix. Leave to cool.
2. Chop the second orange half into pieces and transfer into a bowl. Add in the blueberries, chopped apple and grapes. Pour the cooled tea on top the salad mix and allow to soak a little before serving.
Nutrition: kcal: 200 Net carbs: 40g Fat: 1g Fiber: 5g Protein: 2 g

346. Sirtfood Salmon Lentils Salad
Preparation Time: 10 minutes - **Cooking Time:** 0 minutes - **Servings:** 1
- 20 grams of sliced red onion
- 40 grams of sliced celery
- 10 grams of chopped lovage
- 10 grams of chopped parsley
- Juice of 1/4 of a lemon
- 1 tbsp. of extra virgin olive oil
- 1 large Medjool date, remove pit and chopped
- 1 tbsp. of capers
- 15 grams of chopped walnuts
- 80 grams of avocado, peeled, pitted and sliced
- 100g tinned green lentils or cooked Puy lentils
- 50 grams of chicory leaves
- 50 grams of rocket

1. On a large plate, add the salad leaves.
2. Mix together the remaining ingredients and spread mixture over leaves to serve.
Nutrition: kcal: 400 Net carbs: 20g Fat: 25g Fiber: 14g Protein: 10 g

347. Blueberry Kale Salad with Ginger Lime Dressing
Preparation Time: 10 minutes - **Cooking Time:** 60 minutes - **Servings:** 4
- 3 tbsps. of white wine vinegar
- 1 tbsp. of honey
- 2 tbsps. of finely chopped ginger, crystallized
- 3 tbsps. of lime juice
- Salt and pepper to taste

Salad:
- 1/4 cup of slivered walnuts toasted
- 1/2-3/4 cup of fresh blueberries
- 1/3 thinly sliced red onion
- 8 cups of kale, de-stemmed and chopped into pieces

1. Combine together the entire dressing ingredients in a medium bowl until well mixed.
2. Add sliced onion chopped kale, toss to coat. Leave to marinate for about 1-4 hours, depending on how much time you have, tossing periodically. This is an important step to remove the bitterness from the kale.
3. Add toasted walnuts and blueberries. Toss to coat.
Nutrition: kcal: 91 Net carbs: 10g Fat: 3.69g Fiber: 3g Protein: 3g

348. *Fancy Chicken Salad*
Preparation Time: 1 minute - **Cooking Time:** 10 minutes - **Servings:** 1
- 1 bird's eye chili
- 20 grams of diced red onion
- 1 finely chopped medjool date
- 6 finely chopped Walnut halves
- 100 grams of cooked chicken breast, chopped into bite-sized chunks
- 1/2 tsp of mild curry powder
- 1 tsp of ground turmeric
- 1 tsp of chopped Coriander
- Juice of 1/4 of a lemon
- 75 grams of natural yoghurt
- 40 grams of rocket

1. Mix together the lemon juice in a tub, yoghurt, spices and coriander. Mix in the other ingredients until well blended.
2. Serve over bed of the rocket.
Nutrition: kcal: 340 Net carbs: 22g Fat: 13g Fiber: 5g Protein: 36g

349. *Olive, Tomato, Yellow Pepper, Red Onion, Cucumber Slices and Feta Skewers*
Preparation Time: 5 minutes - **Cooking Time:** 0 minutes - **Servings:** 2
- 100 grams of feta, cut into 8 cubes
- 100 grams of cucumber, cut in quarters and halved Half red onion, cut in half and sliced into 8 pieces
- 1 yellow pepper (or any color you like) cut into 8 squares
- 8 cherry tomatoes
- 8 large black olives
- 2 wooden skewers, soaked for 30 minutes in water before use

For the dressing:
- ½ crushed clove garlic
- 1 tsp of balsamic vinegar
- ½ lemon Juice
- Few finely chopped basil leaves (or ½ tsp of dried mixed herbs)
- 1 tbsp. of extra virgin olive oil
- Few leaves finely chopped oregano (Skip this if using dried mixed herbs)
- Freshly ground black pepper
- Salt to taste

1. Pierce each skewer through the olive, tomato, yellow pepper, red onion, cucumber slices and feta. Repeat a second time.
2. Combine the dressing ingredients in a sealable container and mix thoroughly. Pour dressing over the skewers.
Nutrition: kcal: 228 Net carbs: 13g Fat: 15g Fiber: 3g Protein: 8.7g

350. *Sesame Soy Chicken Salad*
Preparation Time: 10 minutes - **Cooking Time:** 0 minutes - **Servings:** 2
- 150 grams of cooked chicken, shredded Large handful of chopped parsley (20g) ½ finely sliced red onion
- 60 grams of bok choy, very finely shredded
- 100 grams of roughly chopped baby kale
- 1 peeled cucumber, slice in half lengthwise, remove seed and cut into slices
- 1 tbsp. of sesame seeds

For the dressing:
- 2 tsp of soy sauce
- 1 tsp of clear honey
- Juice of 1 lime
- 1 tsp of sesame oil
- 1 tbsp. of extra virgin olive oil

1. Clean your frying pan well and make sure it's dry, toast the sesame seeds for 2 minutes in the pan until fragrant and lightly browned. Set aside in a plate to cool.
2. To Make the Dressing
3. In a small cup, combine the lime juice, soy sauce, olive oil, sesame oil and honey together.
4. Place the kale, cucumber, parsley, red onion and bok choy in a large bowl and mix gently. Pour dressing over salad and mix together.
5. Serve the salad in two different plates and add shredded chicken on top. Just before serving, sprinkle with sesame seeds.
Nutrition: kcal: 304 fat 6 protein 33 carbs 35

Dessert and Snacks

351. *Chocolate Granola*
Preparation time: 10 minutes - **Cooking time:** 38 minutes - **Total time:** 48 minutes - **Servings:** 8
- ¼ cup cacao powder
- ¼ cup maple syrup
- 2 tablespoons coconut oil, melted
- ½ teaspoon vanilla extract
- 1/8 teaspoon salt
- 2 cups gluten-free rolled oats
- ¼ cup unsweetened coconut flakes
- 2 tablespoons chia seeds
- 2 tablespoons unsweetened dark chocolate, chopped finely

1. Preheat your oven to 3000F and use parchment paper to line a medium baking sheet.
2. In a medium pan, add the cacao powder, maple syrup, coconut oil, vanilla extract, and salt, and mix well.
3. Now, over medium heat, position the pan and cook for about 2-3 minutes, or, stirring continuously, until thick and syrupy.
4. Remove from the heat and set aside.
5. Then add the oats, coconut, and chia seeds to a wide bowl and combine well.
6. Add the syrup mixture and mix until well combined.
7. Transfer the granola mixture onto a prepared baking sheet and spread in an even layer.
8. Bake for about 35 minutes.
9. Remove from the oven and leave for around 1 hour to set aside.

10. Add the chocolate pieces and stir to combine.
11. Serve immediately.
Nutrition: Calories 193 Sodium: 24 mg Dietary Fiber: 1.7 g Total Fat: 3.1 g Total Carbs: 16.7 g Protein: 1.5 g

352. *Homemade Marshmallow Fluff*

Preparation time: 10 minutes - Cooking time: 20 minutes - Servings: 2

- 3/4 cup sugar
- 1/2 cup light corn syrup
- 1/4 cup water
- ⅛ teaspoon salt
- 3 little egg whites
- 1/4 teaspoon cream of tartar
- 1 teaspoon 1/2 tsp vanilla extract

1. In a little pan, mix together sugar, corn syrup, salt and water. Attach a candy thermometer into the side of this pan, but make sure it will not touch the underside of the pan.
2. From the bowl of a stand mixer, combine egg whites and cream of tartar. Begin to whip on medium speed with the whisk attachment.
3. Meanwhile, turn a burner on top and place the pan with the sugar mix onto heat. Put the mix into a boil and heat to 240 degrees, stirring periodically.
4. The aim is to have the egg whites whipped to soft peaks and also the sugar heated to 240 degrees at near the same moment. Simply stop stirring the egg whites once they hit soft peaks.
5. Once the sugar has already reached 240 amounts, turn heat low, allowing it to reduce. Insert a little quantity of the popular sugar mix and let it mix. Insert still another little sum of the sugar mix. Add mix slowly and that means you never scramble the egg whites.
6. After all of the sugar was added into the egg whites, then decrease the speed of the mixer and also keep mixing concoction for around 7- 9 minutes until the fluff remains glossy and stiff. At roughly the 5-minute mark, then add the vanilla extract.
7. Use fluff immediately or store in an airtight container in the fridge for around two weeks.
Nutrition: Calories: 159 Sodium: 32 mg Dietary Fiber: 1.5 g Total Fat: 3.1 g Total Carbs: 15.3 g Protein: 1.4 g

353. *Ultimate Chocolate Chip Cookie N' Oreo Fudge Brownie Bar*

Preparation time: 10 minutes - Cooking time: 50 minutes - Servings: 2

- 1 cup (2 sticks) butter, softened
- 1 cup granulated sugar
- 3/4 cup light brown sugar
- 2 large egg
- 1 tablespoon pure vanilla extract
- 2 ½ cups all-purpose flour
- 1 teaspoon baking soda
- 1 teaspoon lemon
- 2 cups (12 oz) milk chocolate chips
- 1 package double stuffed Oreo
- 1 family-size (9×1 3) brownie mixture
- 1/4 cup hot fudge topping

1. Preheat oven to 350 degrees F.
2. Cream the butter and sugar in a wide bowl and use a medium-speed electric mixer for 35 minutes.
3. To blend completely, add the vanilla and eggs and mix well. In another bowl, whisk together the flour, baking soda

and salt, and slowly incorporate in the mixer everything is combined.
4. Stir in chocolate chips.
5. Spread the cookie dough at the bottom of a 9×1-3 baking dish that is wrapped with wax paper and then coated with cooking spray.
6. Shirt with a coating of Oreos. Mix together brownie mix, adding an optional 1/4 cup of hot fudge directly into the mixture.
7. Stir the brownie batter within the cookie-dough and Oreos.
8. Cover with foil and bake at 350 degrees F for 30 minutes.
9. Remove foil and continue baking for another 15 25 minutes.
10. Let cool before cutting on brownies. They may be gooey at the while warm but will also set up perfectly once chilled.
Nutrition: Calories: 145, Sodium: 33 mg, Dietary Fiber: 1.4 g, Total Fat: 4.1 g, Total Carbs: 16.7 g, Protein: 1.3 g.

354. *Crunchy Chocolate Chip Coconut Macadamia Nut Cookies*

Preparation time: 20 minutes - Cooking time: 0 minute - Servings: 2

- 1 cup yogurt
- 1 cup yogurt
- 1/2 teaspoon baking soda
- 1/2 teaspoon salt
- 1 tablespoon of butter, softened
- 1 cup firmly packed brown sugar
- 1/2 cup sugar
- 1 large egg
- 1/2 cup semi-sweet chocolate chips
- 1/2 cup sweetened flaked coconut
- 1/2 cup coarsely chopped dry-roasted macadamia nuts 1/2 cup raisins

1. Preheat the oven to 325°f.
2. Whisk together the rice, oatmeal, baking soda and salt in a small cup, then set aside.
3. In your mixer bowl, mix together the butter/sugar/egg mix.
4. Mix in the flour/oats mix until just combined and stir in the chocolate chips, raisins, nuts, and coconut.
5. Place outsized bits on a parchment-lined cookie sheet.
6. Bake for 1-3 minutes before biscuits are only barely golden brown.
7. Remove from the oven and then leave the cookie sheets to cool at least 10 minutes.
Nutrition: Calories: 167 Sodium: 31 mg Dietary Fiber: 1.4 g Total Fat: 4.1 g Total Carbs: 16.5 g Protein: 1.3 g

355. *Walnut & Date Loaf*

Preparation Time: 10 minutes - Cooking Time: 15 minutes - Servings: 12

- 9 ounces of self-rising flour
- 4 ounces of Medrol dates, chopped
- 2 ounces of walnuts, chopped
- 8fl oz. milk
- 3 eggs
- 1 medium banana, mashed
- 1 teaspoon baking soda

1. In a cup, sieve the baking soda and flour.
2. Add in the banana, eggs, milk and dates and combine all the ingredients thoroughly.
3. Move and smooth out the mixture to a lined loaf tin.
4. Scatter the walnuts on top.

5. Bake the loaf in the oven at 180C/360F for 45 minutes.
Nutrition: Calories: 204 Sodium: 33 mg Dietary Fiber: 1.7 g
Total Fat: 3.1 g Total Carbs: 16.5 g Protein: 1.4 g

356. *Peach and Blueberry Pie*

Preparation time: 1 hour - Cooking time: 0 minute - Servings: 2

- 1 box of noodle dough
- Filling:
- 5 peaches, peeled and chopped (I used roasted peaches)
- 3 cups strawberries
- 3/4 cup sugar
- 1/4 cup bread
- Juice of 1/2 lemon
- 1 egg yolk, beaten

1. Preheat oven to 400 degrees.
2. Place dough to a 9-inch pie plate
3. In a big bowl, combine tomatoes, sugar, bread, and lemon juice, then toss to combine. Pour into the pie plate, mounding at the center.
4. Simply take some of the bread and then cut into bits, then put a pie shirt and put the dough in addition to pressing on the edges.
5. Brush crust with egg wash then sprinkles with sugar.
6. Set onto a parchment paper-lined baking sheet.
7. Cook for about 20 minutes at 400 o'clock, until the crust is browned at the border.
8. Turn oven down to 350, bake for another 40 minutes.
9. Remove and let sit at least 30minutes.
10. Have with vanilla ice-cream.
Nutrition: Calories: 167 Sodium: 31 mg Dietary Fiber: 1.4 g
Total Fat: 4.1 g Total Carbs: 16.6 g Protein: 1.2 g

357. *Pear, Cranberry and Chocolate Crisp*

Preparation time: 10 minutes - Cooking time: 20 minutes - Servings: 3

- Crumble topping:
- 1/2 cup flour
- 1/2 cup brown sugar
- 1 tsp cinnamon
- ⅛ teaspoon salt
- 3/4 cup yogurt
- 1/4 cup sliced peppers
- 1/3 cup butter, melted
- 1 teaspoon vanilla

Filling:
- 1 tablespoon brown sugar
- 3 teaspoons, cut into balls
- 1/4 cup dried cranberries
- 1 teaspoon lemon juice
- Two handfuls of milk chocolate chips

1. Preheat oven to 375.

2. Using butter spray to spray a casserole dish.
3. Put all of the topping ingredients - flour, sugar, cinnamon, salt, nuts, legumes and dried
4. Butter a bowl and then mix. Set aside.
5. Combine the sugar, lemon juice, pears, and cranberries in a wide dish.
6. Once the fully blended move to the prepared baking dish.
7. Spread the topping evenly over the fruit.
8. Bake for about half an hour.
9. Disperse chocolate chips out at the top.

10. Cook for another 10 minutes.
11. Have with ice cream.
Nutrition: Calories: 324 Sodium: 33 mg Dietary Fiber: 1.4 g
Total Fat: 4.1 g Total Carbs: 15.3 g Protein: 1.3 g

358. *Apricot Oatmeal Cookies*

Preparation time: 10 minutes - Cooking time: 20 minutes - Servings: 3

- 1/2 cup (1 stick) butter, softened
- 2/3 cup light brown sugar packed
- 1 egg
- 3/4 cup all-purpose flour
- 1/2 teaspoon baking soda
- 1/2 teaspoon vanilla extract
- 1/2 teaspoon cinnamon
- 1/4 teaspoon salt
- 1 teaspoon 1/2 cups chopped oats
- 3/4 cup yolks
- 1/4 cup sliced apricots
- 1/3 cup slivered almonds
- **Directions:**
- Preheat oven to 350°.

1. In a big bowl, combine with the butter, sugar, and egg until smooth.
2. In another bowl, whisk the flour, baking soda, cinnamon, and salt together.
3. Stir the dry ingredients to the butter-sugar bowl.
4. Now stir in the oats, raisins, apricots, and almonds.
5. I heard on the web that in this time, it's much better to cool with the dough (therefore, your biscuits are thicker)
6. Afterward, I scooped my biscuits into some parchment-lined (easier removal and wash up) cookie sheet - around two inches apart.
7. Sliced mine for approximately ten minutes - they were fantastic!
Nutrition: Calories: 132 Sodium: 33 mg Dietary Fiber: 1.4 g
Total Fat: 3.1 g
Total Carbs: 16.4 g Protein: 1.3 g

359. *Blueberry Muffins*

Preparation time: 15 minutes - Cooking time: 20 minutes - Total time: 35 minutes - Servings: 8

- 1 cup buckwheat flour
- ¼ cup arrowroot starch
- 1½ teaspoons baking powder
- ¼ teaspoon sea salt
- 2 eggs
- ½ cup unsweetened almond milk
- 2–3 tablespoons maple syrup
- 2 tablespoons coconut oil, melted
- 1 cup fresh blueberries

1. Preheat your oven to 3500F and put a muffin tin into 8 cups.
2. In a bowl, place the buckwheat flour, arrowroot starch, baking powder, and salt, and mix well.
3. In a separate bowl, place the eggs, almond milk, maple syrup, and coconut oil, and beat until well combined.
4. Now, place the flour mixture and mix until just combined.
5. Gently, fold in the blueberries.
6. Transfer the mixture into prepared muffin cups evenly.
7. Bake for about 25 minutes or until a toothpick inserted in the center comes out clean.
8. Remove the muffin tin from the oven and position it for about 10 minutes on a wire rack to cool.

9. Carefully invert the muffins onto the wire rack to cool completely before serving.
Nutrition: Calories 136 Sodium: 33 mg Dietary Fiber: 2.4 g Total Fat: 4.5 g Total Carbs: 16.4 g Protein: 1.2 g

360. Chocolate Waffles
Preparation time: 15 minutes - Cooking time: 24 minutes - Total time: 39 minutes - Servings: 8

- 2 cups unsweetened almond milk
- 1 tablespoon fresh lemon juice
- 1 cup buckwheat flour
- ½ cup cacao powder
- ¼ cup flaxseed meal
- 1 teaspoon baking soda
- 1 teaspoon baking powder
- ¼ teaspoons kosher salt
- 2 large eggs
- ½ cup coconut oil, melted
- ¼ cup dark brown sugar
- 2 teaspoons vanilla extract
- 2 ounces unsweetened dark chocolate, chopped roughly

1. Put the almond milk and the lemon juice into a bowl and combine well.
2. Set aside for about 10 minutes.
3. In a bowl, place buckwheat flour, cacao powder, flaxseed meal, baking soda, baking powder, and salt, and mix well.
4. In the bowl of the almond milk mixture, place the eggs, coconut oil, brown sugar, and vanilla extract, and beat until smooth.
5. Now, place the flour mixture and beat until smooth.
6. Gently fold in the chocolate pieces.
7. Preheat and then grease the waffle iron.
8. Place the desired amount of the mixture into the preheated waffle iron and cook for about 3 minutes, or until golden-brown.
9. Repeat with the remaining mixture.
Nutrition: Calories 295 Sodium: 28 mg Dietary Fiber: 1.8 g Total Fat: 3.3 g Total Carbs: 14.2 g Protein: 1.4 g

361. Snowflakes
Preparation time: 10 minutes - Cooking time: 0 minute - Servings: 2

- Won ton wrappers
- Oil for frying
- Powdered sugar

1. Cut won ton wrappers just like you'd a snowflake
2. Heat oil. When hot, add wonton, fry for approximately 30 seconds, then flips over.
3. Drain it with powdered sugar on a paper towel and dust.
Nutrition: Calories: 104 Sodium: 37 mg Dietary Fiber: 1.3 g Total Fat: 4.6 g Total Carbs: 15.6 g Protein: 1.5 g

362. Guilt Totally Free Banana Ice-Cream
Preparation time: 20 minutes - Cooking time: 0 minute - Serves: 3

- 3 quite ripe banana - peeled and chopped A couple of chocolate chips
- 2 tablespoons skim milk

1. In a food processor, throw all ingredients and blend until smooth.
2. Eat: freeze and appreciate afterward.

Nutrition: Calories: 208 Sodium: 33 mg Dietary Fiber: 1.6 g Total Fat: 2.6 g Total Carbs: 14.6 g Protein: 1.8 g

363. Mascarpone Cheesecake With Almond Crust
Preparation time: 10 minutes - Cooking time: 0 minute - Servings: 2
Crust:

- 1/2 cup slivered almonds
- 8 teaspoons or 2/3 cup graham cracker crumbs
- 2 tablespoons sugar
- 1 tablespoon salted butter, melted

Filling:

- 1 (8-ounce) packages cream cheese, room temperature
- 1 (8-ounce) container mascarpone cheese, room temperature 3/4 cup sugar
- 1 teaspoon fresh lemon juice (I needed to use imitation lemon-juice)
- 1 teaspoon vanilla extract
- 2 large eggs, room temperature

1. Preheat the oven to 350 degrees F. For the crust: You're going to need a 9-inch pan (I had a throw off). Finely grind the almonds, sugar in a food processor, cracker crumbs (I used my Magical Bullet). Add the butter and process until they form moist crumbs.
2. Press the almond mixture on the base of the prepared pan (maybe not on the edges of the pan). Bake the crust until it's set and start to brown, about 1-2 minutes. Cool. Minimize the temperature of the oven to 325 degrees F.
3. For your filling: beat the cream cheese, mascarpone cheese, and sugar in a wide bowl with an electric mixer until smooth, sometimes using a rubber spatula to scrape down the sides of the pot. Beat in the vanilla and lemon juice. Add the eggs, one at a time, beating after each addition until combined.
4. Pour the cheese mixture on the crust from the pan. Put the pan into a large skillet or Pyrex bowl, pour the roasting pan with ample hot water to come halfway up the sides of the skillet. Bake for around 1 hour (the dessert can get tough when it's cold) until the center of the filling shifts slightly when the pan is gently shaken. Move to a stand with the cake; cool for 1 hour. Refrigerate for at least eight hours, until the cheesecake is cold.
5. Topping: squeeze just a small thick cream in the microwave using a chopped Lindt dark chocolate afterward, get a Ziplock baggie and cut out a hole at the corner, then pour the melted chocolate into the baggie and used this to decorate the cake!
Nutrition: Calories: 148 Sodium: 26 mg Dietary Fiber: 1.4 g Total Fat: 3.1 g Total Carbs: 11.2 g Protein: 1.6 g

364. Tofu Guacamole
Preparation time: 10 minutes - Cooking time: 30 minutes - Servings: 1

- 8oz silken tofu
- 3 avocados
- 2 tablespoons fresh coriander (cilantro) chopped
- 1 bird's-eye chili
- Juice of 1 lime

1. In a food processor, put all the ingredients and blend a soft chunky consistency with them.
2. Serve with crudités.

Nutrition: Calories: 178 Sodium: 31 mg Dietary Fiber: 1.2 g Total Fat: 4.1 g Total Carbs: 16.6 g Protein: 1.4 g

365. Chocolate Fondue

Preparation Time: 10 minutes - Cooking Time: 15 minutes - Servings: 1

- 4 ounces of dark chocolate min 85% cocoa
- 11 ounces of strawberries
- 7 ounces of cherries
- 2 apples, peeled, cored and sliced
- 3½ FL oz. double cream, heavy cream

1. In a fondue pot or saucepan, place the chocolate and cream then warm it until smooth and creamy.

2. Serve in the fondue pot or transfer it to a serving bowl.
3. Scatter the fruit in a serving dish ready to be dipped into the chocolate.
Nutrition: Calories: 220, Sodium: 43 mg, Dietary Fiber: 5.4 g, Total Fat: 2.1 g, Total Carbs: 1.3 g, Protein: 10.3 g.

366. Choc Nut Truffles

Preparation Time: 10 minutes - Cooking Time: 15 minutes - Servings: 1

- 5 ounces of desiccated shredded coconut
- 2 ounces of walnuts, chopped
- 1 ounce of hazelnuts, chopped
- 4 Medjool dates
- 2 tablespoons 100% cocoa powder or cacao nibs
- 1 tablespoon coconut oil

1. Place ingredients into a blender and process until smooth and creamy.
2. Using a teaspoon, scoop the mixture into bite-size pieces, then roll it into balls.
3. Place them into small paper cases, cover them and chill for 1 hour before serving.
Nutrition: Calories: 220, Sodium: 43 mg, Dietary Fiber: 5.4 g, Total Fat: 2.1 g, Total Carbs: 1.3 g, Protein: 10.3 g.

367. No-Bake Strawberry Flapjacks

Preparation Time: 10 minutes - Cooking Time: 0 minutes - Servings: 1

- 3 ounces of porridge oats
- 4 ounces of dates
- 2 ounces of strawberries
- 2 ounces of peanuts, unsalted
- 2 ounces of walnuts
- 1 tablespoon coconut oil
- 2 tablespoons 100% cocoa powder or cacao nibs

1. Place the ingredients into a blender and process until they become a soft consistency.
2. On a baking sheet or small flat tin, spread the mixture.
3. Press the mixture down and smooth it out.
4. Cut it into 8 pieces, ready to serve.
5. You can add an extra sprinkling of cocoa powder to garnish if you wish.
Nutrition: Calories: 123 Sodium: 30 mg Dietary Fiber: 1.4 g Total Fat: 2.1 g Total Carbs: 11.3 g Protein: 1.3 g

368. Dark Chocolate Pretzel Cookies

Preparation time: 10 minutes - Cooking time: 20 minutes - Servings: 2

- 1 cup yogurt
- 1/2 teaspoon baking soda
- 1/4 teaspoon salt
- 1/4 teaspoon cinnamon
- 4 tablespoons butter (softened/0
- 1/3 cup brown sugar
- 1 egg
- 1/2 teaspoon vanilla
- 1/2 cup dark chocolate chips
- 1/2 cup pretzels, chopped

1. Preheat oven to 350 degrees.
2. Whisk the sugar, butter, vanilla and egg together in a medium dish.
3. In another dish, stir the flour, baking soda, and salt together.
4. Stir the bread mixture in, using all the wet components, along with the chocolate chips and pretzels until just blended.
5. Drop large spoonful of dough on an unlined baking sheet.
6. Bake for 15-17 minutes, or until all of the bottoms are crispy.
7. Allow cooling on a wire rack.
Nutrition: Calories: 150 Sodium: 28 mg Dietary Fiber: 1.7 g Total Fat: 4.1 g Total Carbs: 16.7 g Protein: 1.4 g

369. Matcha With Vanilla

Preparation Time: 5 Minutes - Cooking time: 0 minutes - Servings: 1

Swap the tasty green matcha and the white tea in this Japanese-style tea or coffee. It's easy to make, and it just takes 5 minutes to make it at home.

- Seeds from half a vanilla pod
- ½ teaspoon of matcha powder

1. Heat the kettle, then apply 100ml of water to it. In a tiny cup, pour half the hot water, steam and then transfer the matcha powder and vanilla seeds to the remaining water in the cup.
2. Stir the mixture up to a smooth, slightly smooth and lump-free matcha with a bamboo whisk or mini-electric whisk. In the hot teapot, remove the water and then dump the cooked matcha tea into it. Prefer, with sweet honey or agave.
Nutrition: Calories: 210 Sodium: 34 mg Dietary Fiber: 1.4 g Total Fat: 4.3 g Total Carbs: 15.3 g Protein: 1.6 g

370. Warm Berries & Cream

Preparation Time: 10 minutes - Cooking Time: 15 minutes - Servings: 1

- 9 ounces of blueberries
- 9 ounces of strawberries
- 3 ounces of. Red currants
- 3ounce of blackberries
- Tablespoons fresh whipped cream
- 1 tablespoon honey

1. Mix all ingredients into a bowl.
2. Scoop out a little of the mixture and shape it into a ball.
3. Roll the ball in a little cocoa powder and set aside.
4. Repeat for the remaining mixture. It can be consumed immediately or kept in the fridge.
Nutrition: Calories: 193 Sodium: 32 mg Dietary Fiber: 1.4 g Total Fat: 4.6 g Total Carbs: 16.8 g Protein: 1.6 g

371. Home-Made Ice-Cream Drumsticks

Preparation time: 30 minutes - Cooking time: 0 minute - Servings: 2

- Vanilla ice cream

- Two Lindt hazelnut chunks
- Magical shell - out chocolate
- Sugar levels
- Nuts (I mixed crushed peppers and unsalted peanuts)
- Parchment paper

1. Soften ice cream and mixing topping and two sliced of hazelnut balls.
2. Fill underside of Magic shell with sugar and nuts and top with ice-cream.
3. Wrap parchment paper round cone and then fill cone over about 1.5 inches across the cap of the cone (the paper can help to carry its shape).
4. Sprinkle with magical nuts and shells.
5. Freeze for about 20 minutes, before the ice cream is eaten.
Nutrition: Calories: 153 Sodium: 32 mg Dietary Fiber: 1.4 g Total Fat: 4.1 g Total Carbs: 16.3 g Protein: 1.6 g

372. Mocha Chocolate Mousse

Preparation time: 15 minutes - Cooking time: 2 hours
Dish out s 4-- 6. -
- 250g dark chocolate (85% cocoa solids)
- 6 medium free-range eggs, separated
- 4 table spoon strong black coffee
- 4 table spoon almond milk
- Chocolate coffee beans, to embellish

Melt the chocolate in a big bowl set over a pan of gently simmering water, ensuring the bottom of the bowl does not touch the water. Eliminate the bowl from the first heat and leave the melted chocolate to cool to space temperature level. When the melted chocolate is at space temperature, whisk in the egg yolks one at a time and then carefully fold in the coffee and almond milk.
Using a hand-held electric mixer, blend the egg whites up until stiff peaks form, then blend a couple of tablespoons into the chocolate mixture to loosen it. Carefully fold in the rest, using a big metal spoon.
Transfer the mousse to individual glasses and smooth the surface area. Cover with stick film and chill for a minimum of 2 hours, ideally overnight. Decorate with chocolate coffee beans prior to serving.

373. Best Banana Bread Ever

Preparation time: 15 minutes - Cooking time: 45 minutes
- 150 g unsalted butter melted
- 200 g self-raising flour I utilized brown 1/2 teaspoon bicarbonate of soda 1/2 teaspoon salt
- 150 g light soft brown sugar or caster sugar
- 2 large eggs
- 4 ripe bananas mashed
- 50 g combined seeds or nuts optional

Prefirst heat your microwave oven to 320F.
Place the butter in a little saucepan and melt carefully on a low very first heat. When all the
butter is melted. Turn off and leave to cool for a few minutes.
Line 2 little (1lb) loaf tins with greaseproof paper. Scrunch up a sheet of greaseproof paper big enough to fit in one of your loaf tins. Wet it under the cold tap then utilize it to line the loaf tin.
Repeat with the other tin.
Next, tip the flour into a big bowl and include the bicarbonate of salt, soda and sugar. Stir to integrate.

Peel the bananas and rip them into pieces. Location the banana chunks in a small bowl or
container. Utilize a potato masher to mash them approximately then include the eggs and stir to combine.
Idea the eggs and banana mix into the dry things r eq uired and stir completely up until you have a thick batter. Consist of the cooled melted butter and stir well.
Consist of the nuts or seeds, if you are utilizing them, and stir as soon as more till the seeds are uniformly dispersed.
Divide the mix between the 2 loaf tins and cook the banana bread in your prefirst heated
microwave oven for 45 minutes. If not prepare your banana bread for a more 5 minutes and
examine again.
When your banana bread is prepared. Eliminate from the microwave oven. Allow to cool for 5 minutes then remove from the tin, peel off the greaseproof paper and cool on a cake rack ... or enjoy while it is still warm!

374. Raw Brownie Bites

Preparation time: 2,50 hours
- Whole walnuts 2½ cups
- Almonds ¼ cup
- Medjool dates 2½ cups
- Cacao powder 1 cup
- Vanilla extract one teaspoon
- Sea salt ⅛-¼ teaspoon

Place all once well mixed in a food processor.
Place on a baking sheet and freeze for 30 minutes, or 2 hours in the refrigerator. Roll yourself into balls.

375. Avocado Mayo Medley

Preparation time: 5 minutes - Cooking time: 0 minutes - Servings: 3
- 1 medium avocado, cut into chunks
- ½ teaspoon ground cayenne pepper
- 2 tablespoons fresh cilantro ¼ cup olive oil
- ½ cup mayo, low fat and los sodium

Take a food processor and add avocado, cayenne pepper, lime juice, salt and cilantro.
Mix until smooth.
Slowly incorporate olive oil add 1 tablespoon at a time and keep processing between additions. Store and use as needed!

376. Hearty Almond Crackers

Preparation time: 10 minutes - Cooking Time: 20 minutes
- 1 cup almond flour
- ¼ teaspoon of baking soda and 1/8 teaspoon of black pepper
- 3 tablespoons sesame seeds
- 1 egg, beaten
- Salt and pepper to taste

Preheat to 350 degrees F in your oven.
Line two parchment paper baking sheets and hold them on one side.
Break the dough into 2 balls.
Roll the dough in between two parchment paper bits.
Break the crackers and pass them on to the baking sheet that has been prepared.
For 15-20 minutes, bake.
Repeat until all of the dough has been used up.
Leave crackers to cool and serve.

377. Black Bean Salsa

Preparation time: 5 minutes - Cooking time: 0 minutes - Servings: 3

- 1 tablespoon coconut aminos
- ½ teaspoon cumin, ground
- 1 cup canned black beans, no salt
- 1 cup of salsa
- 6 cups romaine lettuce, torn
- ½ cup avocado, peeled, pitted and cubed

Take a bowl and add beans, alongside other ingredients.
Toss well and serve.

378. Corn Spread

Preparation time: 5 minutes - Cooking time: 0 minutes - Servings: 3

- 30 ounce canned corn, drained
- 2 green onions, chopped
- ½ cup coconut cream
- 1 jalapeno, chopped
- ½ teaspoon chili powder

Take a pan and add corn, green onions, jalapeno, chili powder, stir well.
Bring to a simmer over medium heat and cook for 10 minutes.
Let it chill and add coconut cream.
Stir well.

379. Special Green Tea Smoothie

Preparation time: 10 Minutes - Cooking Time: 0 minutes - Servings 2

- 250 ml milk
- 2 ripe bananas
- 1/2 tsp vanilla bean paste
- 2 teaspoons of honey
- 6 ice cubes
- 2 teaspoons of matcha green tea powder

Using a blender or smoothie machine, combine all the ingredients together. Enjoy and serve.

380. Special Blackcurrant and Oat Yoghurt

Preparation time: 10 Minutes - Cooking Time: 0 Minutes - Servings 4

- 400 grams of greek yogurt, plain
- 200g blackcurrants, washed and stalks removed
- 200 ml of water
- 4 tablespoon of caster sugar (or your own choice of sweetener)
- 80 grams of oats

In a small pan, simply place the blackcurrants, water, and sugar. Bring to boil.
After boiling, slightly reduce the heat, maintain the simmer and cook for another 4 to 5 minutes.
Turn off the heat and allow it to cool the mixture.
After cooling, you can now refrigerate your blackcurrant compote until ready to be used.
Using a large bowl, place the yogurt and oats, then thoroughly stir in together.
Divide the blackcurrant compote into 4 serving bowls, then just a simple top with the oats and yogurt. Mix and enjoy.

381. Fruit & Nut Yoghurt Crunch

Preparation time: 5 minutes - Cooking time: 25 minutes - Servings: 4

- 100g (3½ oz) plain Greek yogurt
- 50g (2oz) strawberries, chopped
- 6 walnut halves, chopped
- Sprinkling of cocoa powder

1. Stir half of the chopped strawberries into the yogurt.
2. Using a glass, place a layer of yogurt with a sprinkling of strawberries and walnuts,
followed by another layer of the same until you reach the top of the glass.
3. Garnish with walnuts pieces and a dusting of cocoa powder.

382. Fruity Granola Bars

Preparation time: 5 minutes - Cooking time: 30 minutes - Servings: 3

- ¾ cup packed brown sugar ½ cup honey
- ¼ cup water
- 1 teaspoon salt
- ½ cup cocoa butter 3 cups rolled oats
- 1 cup walnuts, chopped
- 1 cup ground buckwheat ¼ cup sesame seeds
- ½ cup dried strawberries or mixed fruits ½ cup raisins
- ½ cup Medjool dates, chopped

In a large pan, combine sugar, cocoa butter, honey, water, and salt. Bring to a simmer and cook for 5 minutes.
Score deeply into bars roughly 2" wide by 4" tall.
Allow cooling for 30 minutes before breaking or cutting along score lines. Store in an airtight container.

383. Cardamom Granola Bars

Preparation time: 5 minutes - Cooking time: 30 minutes - Servings: 3

- 2 cups rolled oats
- ½ cup raisins
- ½ cup walnuts, chopped and toasted
- 1 ½ teaspoon ground cardamom
- 6 tablespoons cocoa butter 1/3 cup packed brown sugar 3 tablespoons honey Coconut oil, for greasing pan

Preheat the oven to 350°F.
With foil, line a 9-inch square pan, spreading the foil over the edges. Grease the coconut oil on the foil.
Mix the oats, raisins, walnuts and cardamom in a large bowl.
Heat the cocoa butter, brown sugar and honey in a saucepan until the butter melts and begins to bubble.
Bake on top for approximately 30 minutes or until golden brown.
Enable it to cool for 30 minutes. With the foil, lift the granola out of the pan, place the cutting board on and put it on. Cut into 18 bars.

384. Coconut Brownie Bites

Preparation time: 5 minutes - Cooking time: 40 minutes - Servings: 3

- ¼ cup unsweetened cocoa powder
- ¼ cup unsweetened desiccated or shredded coconut

In a food processor, put everything and blend until well combined.
Roll into 1" balls.

Roll balls in coconut until well-covered and place on a wax paper-lined baking sheet.
Freeze for 30 minutes or refrigerate for up to 2 hours.

385. Tortilla Chips and Fresh Salsa
Preparation time: 5 minutes - Cooking time: 50 minutes - Servings: 3
* 4 whole wheat flour tortillas
* 2 tablespoons extra virgin olive oil
* 4 Roma tomatoes, diced
* 1 small red onion, finely diced
* 1 Bird's Eye chili pepper, finely diced
* 2 teaspoons parsley, finely chopped
* 2 teaspoons cilantro, finely chopped
* 1 lime, juiced
* Salt and pepper to taste

Preheat oven to 350 degrees F.
Cover one side of each tortilla in olive oil using a pastry brush.
Divide each tortilla into 8 wedges with a sharp knife or pizza cutter. Spread the tortillas in a single layer over a large baking sheet. If possible, use more than one baking sheet.
Bake for 8 to 10 minutes, until both sides are golden brown and your chips are crispy, flipping halfway through.
While the chips are baking, combine tomatoes, red onion, chili pepper, parsley, cilantro and lime juice and mix well.
Serve salsa with the chips.

386. The Bell Pepper Fiesta
Preparation time: 5 minutes - Cooking time: 0 minutes - Servings: 3
* 2 tablespoons dill, chopped
* 1 yellow onion, chopped
* 1 pound multicolored peppers, cut, halved, seeded and cut into thin strips
* 3 tablespoons organic olive oil
* 2 ½ tablespoons white wine vinegar
* Black pepper to taste

Take a bowl and mix in sweet pepper, onion, dill, pepper, oil, vinegar and toss well.
Divide between bowls and serve.

387. Spiced Up Pumpkin Seeds Bowls
Preparation time: 5 minutes - Cooking time: 30 minutes - Servings: 3
* ½ tablespoon chili powder
* ½ teaspoon cayenne
* 2 cups pumpkin seeds
* 2 teaspoons lime juice

Spread pumpkin seeds over a lined baking sheet, add lime juice, cayenne and chili powder.Toss well.
Preheat your oven to 275 degrees F.
Roast in your oven for 20 minutes and transfer to small bowls.

388. Mozzarella Cauliflower Bars
Preparation time: 5 minutes - Cooking time: 30 minutes - Servings: 3
* 1 cauliflower head, riced
* 12 cup low-fat mozzarella cheese, shredded ¼ cup egg whites
* 1 teaspoon Italian dressing, low fat
* Pepper to taste

Spread over a lined baking sheet with cauliflower rice.
Preheat your oven to 375 degrees F.
Roast for 20 minutes.
Transfer to bowl and spread pepper, cheese, seasoning, egg whites and stir well.
Spread in a rectangular pan and press.
Transfer to the oven and cook for an additional 20 minutes.

389. Feta and Beet Stacked Appetizer
Preparation time: 5 minutes - Cooking time: 20 minutes - Servings: 4
* 2 large fresh beets
* ½ teaspoon dried lovage
* ½ cup red wine vinegar
* ¼ cup lemon juice (optional) ½ cup feta cheese
* ½ cup walnuts, crushed

Soak the lovage in the red wine vinegar while you're preparing the rest of the appetizer.
Bring a pot of water to a boil and cook the beets for 25 minutes or until they are tender.
Cool, peel, and slice in 1/3" thick slices.
Place beets in a bowl with the lovage red wine vinegar and marinate 15 minutes.
Separate the beets from the vinegar and add the lemon juice to the liquid. Place a few beet slices on a microwave-safe dish and sprinkle them with some feta cheese and crushed walnuts. Drizzle with some of the lemon vinegar mixes.
Top with more beet slices, and sprinkle again with feta, walnuts and lemon vinegar. Repeat until you have no more beet slices left.
Microwave for 45 seconds to 1 minute on medium.
Cool slightly before serving.

390. Blueberry Nut Bran Muffins
Preparation time: 5 minutes - Cooking time: 10 minutes - Servings: 4
* Wheat bran – 1 cup
* Whole wheat flour – 1.5 cups
* Sea salt - .5 teaspoon
* Baking soda - .25 teaspoon
* Baking powder - .25 teaspoon
* Cinnamon – 1.5 teaspoons
* Eggs – 2
* Soy milk, unsweetened - .75 cup
* Apple cider vinegar – 1 tablespoon
* Apple sauce, unsweetened - .33 cup
* Date sugar – .5 cup
* Soybean oil - .33 cup
* Blueberries, fresh or frozen – 1 cup
* Walnuts, chopped - .5 cup

Begin by setting your standard or toaster oven to Fahrenheit four-hundred degrees. Line a twelve-cup muffin tin and then spray the paper liners with nonstick cooking spray.
Whisk together the eggs, applesauce, date sugar, soybean oil, soy milk, and apple cider vinegar in a large bowl until fully combined. Set it aside.
In another clean cup, whisk together the whole wheat flour, wheat bran, cinnamon, sea salt, baking soda, and baking soda. Once the dry ingredients are combined, fol them into the other prepared ingredients. Gently fold in the blueberries and walnuts, just until combined.
Divide the blueberry nut bran muffin batter between the prepared muffin liners and allow them to cook until fully done and a toothpick once inserted is removed clean, about

fifteen to eighteen minutes. Enable the muffins to cool for five minutes before removing them from the oven. Withdrawing them from the pan.

391. Plum Oat Bars

Preparation time: 5 minutes - Cooking time: 10 minutes - Servings: 4
- Rolled oats – 1.5 cups
- Baking powder – 1 teaspoon
- Almond meal - .5 cup
- Cinnamon – 1.5 teaspoon
- Soybean oil – 2 tablespoons
- Sea salt - .25 teaspoon
- Prunes – 2 cups

Begin by preheating the oven to Fahrenheit three-hundred and fifty degrees and preparing the prunes. Add the prunes to a large bowl and pour hot water over them until fully submerged.

Allow the prunes to sit in the water for five minutes, until soft.

Remove the prunes from the water and transfer them to a blender or food processor, reserving the water. Pour in a small amount of the water that you previously reserved from the prunes and blend until the prunes form a thick paste.

Add two tablespoons of the prepared prune puree to a medium kitchen bowl along with the oil, sea salt, baking powder, cinnamon, almond flour, and rolled oats. Combine together until the mixture resembles a crumble, slightly like wet sand. You can add more prune puree if it is too dry.

Line a square baking dish with kitchen parchment and then press three-quarters of the oat mixture into the bottom to form a crust. Spread the remaining prune puree over the top of the crust, and then sprinkle the remaining oat mixture over the prune puree to add a crumble.

Cook the bars in the oven until set and slightly toasted, about fifteen minutes. Remove the plum oat bars from the hot oven and let the pan cool completely. After the bars have reached room temperature slice them into nine bars and enjoy.

392. Spinach and Kale Mix

Preparation time: 5 minutes - Cooking time: 30 minutes - Servings: 4
- 2 chopped shallots
- 1 c. no-salt-added and chopped canned tomatoes
- 2 c. baby spinach
- 2 minced garlic cloves
- 5 c. torn kale
- 1 tbsp. olive oil

Heat up a pan with the oil over medium-high heat, add the shallots, stir and sauté for 5 minutes.

Add the spinach, kale and the other ingredients, toss, cook for 10 minutes more, divide between plates and serve.

393. Kale Dip with Cajun Pita Chips

Preparation time: 10 minutes - Baking time: 8 – 10 minutes - Cooling time: 1 hour
For the Dip:
- 2 cups sour cream
- 1 ½ cups baby kale
- ¼ cup red bell pepper, diced
- ¼ cup green onions, diced
- 1 clove garlic, minced
- 1/8 teaspoon chili pepper flakes

For the Chips:
- 5 pita bread, halved and split open
- ½ cup extra virgin olive oil
- ½ teaspoon Cajun seasoning ¼ teaspoon ground cumin ¼ teaspoon turmeric
- Salt to taste

To make the dip: In a bowl, combine the sour cream, baby kale, red pepper, onions, garlic, salt and chili pepper flakes. Cover and refrigerate for at least 1 hour. For the processing of chips: Preheat the oven to 400 degrees F.

Break half of each pita into four wedges. Combine the Cajun seasoning, olive oil, cumin and turmeric and brush over the rough side of the wedges of the pita. Place on ungreased baking sheets and cook for 8-10 minutes or until golden brown and crisp chips are available.

Serve with dip.

394. Snack Bites

Preparation Time: 5 Minutes - Cooking time: 35 Minutes - Servings: 2
- 120g walnuts
- 30g dark chocolate (85% cocoa)
- 250g dates
- 1 tablespoon pure cocoa powder
- 1 tablespoon turmeric
- 1 tablespoon of olive oil

Contents of a pod of vanilla or other flavoring of vanilla Coarsely crumble the chocolate and mix it with the walnuts in a food
processor into a fine powder.

Then add the other ingredients and stir until you have a uniform dough. If necessary, add 1 to 2 tablespoons of water.

Form 15 pieces from the mixture and refrigerate in an airtight tin for at least one hour.

The bites will remain in the refrigerator for a week.

395. Spinach Mix

Preparation time: 10 minutes - Cooking time: 12 minutes - Servings: 4
- 1 pound baby spinach
- 1 yellow onion, chopped
- 1 tablespoon olive oil
- 1 tablespoon lemon juice
- 2 garlic cloves, minced
- A pinch of cayenne pepper
- ¼ teaspoon smoked paprika

Heat up a pan with the oil over medium-high heat, add the onion and the
garlic and sauté for 2 minutes.

Add the cooked spinach for 10 minutes over medium heat, divide between
Plates and as a side dish to eat.

396. Walnut Stuffed Bacon Wrapped Dates

Preparation time: 10 - 20minutes - Baking time: 10 minutes - Servings: 4
- 4 ounces walnuts, halved

Preheat your broiler.

Slit the dates and place one walnut half inside each. Wrap dates with ½ slice of bacon, using
toothpicks to hold them together.

Broil 10 minutes, turning once, or until bacon is evenly brown and crisp.

397. Loaded Chocolate Fudge

Preparation time: 10 minutes - Cooking Time: 1+ hours
- 1 cup Medjool dates, chopped
- 2 tablespoons coconut oil, melted
- 1/2 cup peanut butter
- ¼ cup of unsweetened cocoa powder ½ cup walnuts
- 1 teaspoon vanilla

Lightly grease an 8' square baking pan with coconut oil and soak the dates in warm water for 20-30 minutes.

Add dates, peanut butter, cocoa powder and vanilla to a food processor and blend until smooth. Fold in walnuts.

Pack into the greased baking pan and put in your freezer for 1 hour or until

fudge is solid and firm.

Cut into 16 or more bite-sized squares and store in semi-airtight container in the refrigerator.

398. Kale Chips

Preparation Time: 5 Minutes - Cooking time: 55 Minutes - Servings: 2
- 1 large head of curly kale, wash, dry and pulled from stem 1 tbsp. extra virgin
- olive oil
- Minced parsley
- A squeeze of lemon juice
- Cayenne pepper (just a pinch)
- Dash of soy sauce

In a large bowl, rip the kale from the stem into palm-sized pieces. Sprinkle the minced parsley, olive oil, soy sauce, a squeeze of the lemon juice, and a very small pinch of the cayenne powder.

Toss with a set of tongs or salad forks, and make sure to coat all of the leaves.

If you have a dehydrator, turn it on to 118 F, spread out the kale on a dehydrator sheet, and leave in there for about 2 hours.

If you are cooking them, place parchment paper on top of a cookie sheet. Lay the bed of kale and separate it a bit to make sure the kale is evenly toasted. Cook for 10-15 minutes maximum at 250F.

399. Moroccan Leeks Snack

Preparation time: 5 minutes - Cooking time: 0 minutes - Servings: 3
- 1 bunch radish, sliced
- 3 cups leeks, chopped
- 1 ½ cups olives, pitted and sliced
- Pinch turmeric powder
- 2 tablespoons essential olive oil
- 1 cup cilantro, chopped

Take a bowl and mix in radishes, leeks, olives and cilantro. Mix well.

Season with pepper, oil, turmeric and toss well.

400. Honey Nuts

Preparation Time: 5 Minutes - Cooking time: 35 Minutes - Servings: 2
- 150g (5oz) walnuts

- 150g (5oz) pecan nuts
- 50g (2oz) softened butter
- 1 tablespoon honey
- ½ bird's-eye chili, very finely chopped and deseeded

Preheat the 180C/360F oven. In a cup, mix the butter, honey and chili and add the nuts and stir well. Spread the nuts over a lined baking sheet and roast for 10 minutes in the oven, stirring halfway through once. Take it out of the oven and allow it to cool before eating.

401. Pear, Cranberry and Chocolate Crisp

Preparation Time: 15 Minutes - Cooking Time: 10 Minutes - Servings: 10
- 1/2 cup flour
- 1/2 cup brown sugar
- 1 tsp. cinnamon
- 1/8 tsp. salt
- 3/4 cup yogurt
- 1/4 cup sliced peppers
- 1/3 cup butter, melted
- 1 teaspoon vanilla

Filling:
- 1 tbsp. brown sugar
- 1/4 cup dried cranberries
- 1 teaspoon of lemon juice
- Two handfuls of milk chocolate chips

1. Preheat oven to 375.
2. Using butter spray to spray a casserole dish.
3. Put all of the topping **ingredients** — flour, sugar, cinnamon, salt, nuts, etc.
4. Butter a bowl and then mix. Set aside.
5. Combine the sugar, lemon juice, pears and cranberries in a big cup.
6. Once is fully blended, move to the prepared baking dish.
7. Spread the topping evenly over the fruit.
8. Bake for about half an hour.
9. Disperse chocolate chips out at the top.
10. Cook for another 10 minutes.
11. Have with ice cream.
Nutrition: Calories: 128 Cal Fat: 6.6 g Carbs: 15 g Fiber: 0.7 g Protein: 2 g

402. Radish green pesto

Preparation Time: 15 Minutes - Cooking Time: 60 Minutes - Servings: 10
- 2 handfuls
- fresh radish leaf (from 1–2 bunch of radishes in organic quality) 1 garlic
- 30 g pine nuts (2 tbsp)
- 30 g parmesan (1 piece; 30% fat in dry matter)
- 100 ml olive oil
- salt
- pepper
- 1 tsp lemon juice

1. Wash the radish leaves and shake them dry. Peel and chop the garlic.
2. Roast pine nuts in a hot pan without fat over medium heat for 3 minutes. Grate the Parmesan finely.
3. Puree the radish leaves, garlic, pine nuts and the oil with a hand blender. Mix in the Parmesan. Season with salt, pepper and lemon juice.

403. Watercress smoothie

Preparation Time: 15 Minutes - **Cooking Time:** 60 Minutes - **Servings:** 10

- 150 g watercress
- 1 small onion
- ½ cucumber
- 1 tbsp lemon juice
- 200 ml mineral water
- salt
- pepper
- 4 tbsp crushed ice

1. Wash and spin dry watercress; put some sheets aside for the garnish.
2. The onion should be peeled and cut into small cubes. Wash the cucumber half, halve lengthways and cut the pulp into tiny cubes; Set aside 4 tablespoons of cucumber cubes.
3. Puree the remaining cucumber cubes with cress, onion cubes, lemon juice, mineral water and ice in a blender.
4. Season the smoothie with salt and pepper, pour into 2 glasses and sprinkle with cucumber cubes and cress leaves.

404. Melon and spinach juice with cinnamon

Preparation Time: 15 Minutes - **Cooking Time:** 60 Minutes - **Servings:** 10

- 350 g small honeydew melon (0.5 small honeydew melons)
- 250 g young tender spinach leaves
- 1 PC cinnamon stick (approx. 1 cm)
- nutmeg

1. Core the melon with a teaspoon. First cut the melon into wedges, then cut the pulp from the skin and roughly dice.
2. Clean the spinach and wash thoroughly in a bowl of water. Renew the water several times until it remains clear.
3. Using a small sharp knife, scrape thin strips off the cinnamon stick.
4. Squeeze the spinach lightly; Put back a leaflet and a small stem for the garnish as you like. Juice the rest with the melon in a juicer and pour it into a glass with ice cubes. Rub a little nutmeg over it, garnish with cinnamon and possibly with the spinach set aside.

405. Christmas cocktail - vegan eggnog

- 1 cup cashew nuts
- 1 cup soy or almond milk
- 2-3 glasses of water
- about 5 pieces of dates (more if you like sweeter drinks)
- 2-3 scoops of brandy or whiskey
- 1 tablespoon lemon juice (optional, to taste)
- 1-2 teaspoons cinnamon
- ½ teaspoons ground anise
- ½ teaspoons ground ginger
- 2 pinches nutmeg
- pinch of salt

1. Pour dates and cashews with boiling water and leave to soak for 20 minutes. Transfer the remaining ingredients to the blender dish and finally add the drained nuts and dates.
2. Mix thoroughly in a high-speed blender for a few minutes, until a thick and creamy cocktail without lumps is formed. If your blender can't do it, mix the cashews with water first and strain them with gauze.

3. Season the cocktail with more lemon juice and salt to tasteand if you prefer sweeter drinks, add 2-3 pieces of dates. Serve it chilled with a pinch of cinnamon.

406. Orange and mandarin liqueur

Preparation Time: 15 Minutes - **Cooking Time:** 60 Minutes - **Servings:** 10

- 2 large oranges
- 2 tangerines
- 1 small lemon
- 300 g white sugar candy
- 1 stick of vanilla
- 50 ml of orange juice
- 250 ml double grain

1. Put the sugar candy in a bottle or a screw-top jar.
2. Pour the citrus into small pieces and remove the skin.
3. Pour in the orange juice.
4. Add the vanilla stick.
5. Baste with the double grain.
6. Fill up to the top of the bottle if desired.
7. Close the bottle.
8. Shake daily until the sugar candy has dissolved.
9. After 2 - 3 weeks pour the liqueur through a sieve.
10. Pour it back into the bottle.

407. Cucumber-apple-banana shake

Preparation Time: 15 Minutes - **Cooking Time:** 60 Minutes - **Servings:** 10

- 1 lemon
- 1 banana
- 4th sour apples (e.g. granny smith)
- 1 bunch parsley
- ½ cucumber
- mineral water to fill up
- 10 dice ice cubes

1. Break the lemon in half and suck the juice out. Peel and dice the banana. Clean, wash, quarter the apples, remove the core, dice the pulp. Mix the apples with the banana cubes and lemon juice.
2. Wash parsley, shake dry and chop. Clean, peel and halve the cucumber, coreand cut into bite-size pieces. Put 3 pieces of cucumber on 4 wooden skewers.
3. Puree the remaining pieces of cucumber with fruit, parsley and ice in a blender. Spread over 4 glasses, fill up with mineral water to the desired consistency and garnish with 1 cucumber skewer each.

408. Kefir avocado shake with herbs

Preparation Time: 15 Minutes - **Cooking Time:** 60 Minutes - **Servings:** 10

- 2 stems dill
- 2 stems parsley
- straws of chives
- 1 avocado
- 1 tsp honey
- 1 splash lime juice
- 4 ice cubes
- 300 ml kefir chilled
- salt
- 1 pinch wasabi powder

1. Spray the herbs, pat dry, pluck and cut roughly except for a few dill tips for the garnish.

2. Peel, halve, core and cut the avocado into pieces. Puree with the herbs, honey, lime juice, ice cubes and kefir in a blender until creamy.
3. Season the smoothie with salt and wasabi and pour into glasses. Serve garnished with dill tips.

409. Mandarin liqueur
Preparation Time: 15 Minutes - **Cooking Time:** 60 Minutes - **Servings:** 10
- 2 large oranges
- 2 tangerines
- 1 small lemon
- 300 g white sugar candy
- 1 stick of vanilla
- 50 ml of orange juice
- 250 ml double grain

1. Put the sugar candy in a bottle or a screw-top jar.
2. Pour the citrus into small pieces and remove the skin.
3. Pour in the orange juice.
4. Add the vanilla stick.
5. Baste with the double grain and fill up to the top of the bottle if desired.
6. Close the bottle.
7. Shake daily until the sugar candy has dissolved.
8. After 2 - 3 weeks pour the liqueur through a sieve and pour it back into the bottle.

410. Pear and lime marmalade
Ingredients for 1.5 l jam
- 3-4 untreated limes
- 1 kg ripe pears
- 500 g jam sugar 2: 1

1. Wash 2 limes and grate dry.
2. Peel the peels thinly with the zest ripper.
3. Then cut all limes in half and squeeze them out. Measure out100 ml of lime juice.
4. Wash and peel the pears, remove the core and then quarter them. Weigh 900 g of pulp.
5. Then puree the pears together with the lime juice.
6. Now put the pear puree together with the lime peels and the jellied sugar in a saucepan.
7. Bring all **ingredients** to the boil together.
8. Simmer for 4 minutes, stirring, taking care not to burn anything.
9. Make a gelation test with a small blob on a cold saucer. If this becomes solid in a short time, the jam is ready.
10. Remove any foam that may have formed with a spade, but you can also simply stir it in.
11. Then pour the hot mass into hot rinsed jars, close and let stand upside down.

411. Healthy green shot
Preparation Time: 15 Minutes - **Cooking Time:** 60 Minutes - **Servings:** 10
- 2 pears
- 3 green apples (e.g. granny smith)
- 3 sticks celery
- 60 g organic ginger
- 1 bunch parsley (20 g)
- 3 kiwi fruit
- 2 limes
- 1 tsp turmeric

1. Wash pears, apples, celery, ginger and parsley and cut into pieces. Halve the kiwi fruit and remove the pulp with a spoon. Halve limes and squeeze out juice.
2. Put the pears, apples, kiwi, celery, ginger and parsley in the juicer and squeeze out the juice.
3. Mix freshly squeezed juice with the lime juice and season with turmeric. Serve the mixture as shots immediately or freeze it in portions.

412. Spinach kiwi smoothie bowl
Preparation Time: 15 Minutes - **Cooking Time:** 60 Minutes - **Servings:** 10
- 1 green apple
- 2 kiwi fruit
- 300 g bananas (2 bananas)
- 100 g baby spinach
- 1 lemon
- 6 g chia seeds (2 tsp)
- 20 g grated coconut (2 tbsp)

1. Clean, wash, core and chop the apple. Peel and cut the kiwis and bananas and put half aside. Wash the spinach and put some leaves aside. Halve the lemon and squeeze out the juice.
2. Put half of the fruit, spinach and lemon juice in a blender and mash finely. Divide the smoothie into 4 bowls.
3. Put the remaining pieces of fruit as a topping on the smoothie bowls. Sprinkle with chia seeds and grated coconut and serve with the remaining spinach leaves.

413. Avocado smoothie with basil
Preparation Time: 15 Minutes - **Cooking Time:** 60 Minutes - **Servings:** 10
- 2 kiwi fruit
- 1 yellow-peeled apple
- 200 g honeydew melon meat
- 1 avocado
- 1 green chili pepper
- 20 g basil (1 handful)
- 20 g arugula (0.25 bunch)
- 1 tbsp sprouts (suitable for raw consumption)

1. Peel and slice the kiwi fruit. Clean the apple, quarter and core it and break the quarters into slices. Cut the melon meat into pieces. Peel, core and cut avocado into pieces. Wash the chili pepper and cut it into rings. Wash the basil and rocket and shake dry. Shower sprouts in a sieve.
2. Put all prepared **ingredients** in a blender and mash them finely. Add about 100 ml of cold water and serve in 4 glasses.

414. Blackberry and vanilla smoothie
Preparation Time: 15 Minutes - **Cooking Time:** 60 Minutes - **Servings:** 10
- 500 g blackberry
- 1 vanilla bean
- 1 tsp lemon juice
- 700 ml buttermilk (ice cold)
- 80 g lean quark (4 tbsp)
- 40 g cashews
- 80 ml whipped cream

1. Wash and drain blackberries.
2. Cut the length of the vanilla pod, scrape the creamy pulp and puree in a blender with blackberries, lemon juice, buttermilk, curd cheese and cashew nuts.

3. Whip the cream. Pour smoothie into 4 glasses and garnish with cream

415. *Dijon Celery Salad*

Preparation Time: 10 minutes - **Cooking Time:** 0 minutes - **Servings:** 4

- 5 teaspoons stevia
- ½ cup lemon juice
- 1/3 cup dijon mustard
- 2/3 cup olive oil
- black pepper to the taste
- 2 apples, cored, peeled and cubed
- 1 bunch celery and leaves, roughly chopped ¾ cup walnuts, chopped

1. In a salad bowl, mix celery and its leaves with apple pieces and walnuts.
2. Add black pepper, lemon juice, mustard, stevia and olive oil.
3. Whisk well, add to your salad, toss.
4. Divide into small cups and serve as a snack.
Nutrition: Calories: 125 Cal Fat: 2 g Carbohydrates: 7 g Protein: 7 g Fiber: 2 g

416. *Dill Bell Pepper Snack Bowls*

Preparation Time: 10 minutes - **Cooking Time:** 0 minutes - **Servings:** 4

- 2 tablespoons dill, chopped
- 1 yellow onion, chopped
- 1-pound multicolored bell peppers, cut into halves, seeded and cut into thin strips
- 3 tablespoons olive oil
- 2 and ½ tablespoons white vinegar
- Black pepper to the taste

1. In a salad bowl, mix bell peppers with onion, dill, pepper, oil and vinegar, toss to coat, divide into small bowls and serve as a snack.
Nutrition: Calories: 120 Cal Fat: 3 g Carbohydrates: 2 g Protein: 3 g Fiber: 3 g

417. *Cinnamon Apple Chips*

Preparation Time: 10 minutes - **Cooking Time:** 2 hours - **Servings:** 4

- Cooking spray
- 2 teaspoons cinnamon powder
- 2 apples, cored and thinly sliced

On a lined baking sheet, arrange the apple slices, sprinkle with cooking oil, sprinkle with cinnamon, place in the oven and cook at 300 degrees F for 2 hours.
Divide and serve as a snack in bowls.
Nutrition: Calories: 80 Cal Fat: 0 g Carbohydrates: 7 g Protein: 4 g Fiber: 3 g

418. *Herb Roasted Chickpeas*

Preparation time: 5 minutes - **Cooking time:** 30 minutes - **Servings:** 3

- 1 can of chickpeas, drained
- 1 - 2 tablespoon extra-virgin olive oil
- ½ teaspoon dried lovage
- ½ teaspoon dried basil
- 1 teaspoon garlic powder
- 1/8 teaspoon cayenne powder
- ¼ teaspoon fine salt

Preheat the oven to 400 degrees F and use parchment paper to cover a large baking sheet.
Spread chickpeas out evenly over the pan in a single layer and roast for 30 minutes.
Remove from oven and transfer to a heat-resistant bowl.
Add the olive oil and toss to coat each chickpea. Sprinkle with herbs and toss again to distribute.
Return to oven for an additional 15 minutes.
Until eating, let it cool for at least 15 minutes.

419. *Beans Snack Salad*

Preparation Time: 10 minutes - **Cooking Time:** 0 minutes - **Servings:** 6

- 2 cups tomatoes, chopped
- 2 cups cucumber, chopped
- 3 cups mixed greens
- 2 cups mung beans, sprouted
- 2 cups clover sprouts

for the salad dressing:

- 1 tablespoon cumin, ground
- 1 cup dill, chopped
- 4 TABLESPOONS LEMON JUICE
- 1 avocado, pitted, peeled and roughly chopped
- 1 cucumber, roughly chopped

1. In a salad bowl.
2. Mix tomatoes with 2 cups cucumber, greens, clover and mung sprouts.
3. In your blender, mix cumin with dill, lemon juice, 1 cucumber and avocado.
4. Blend well, add this to your salad, toss well and serve as a snack.
Nutrition: Calories: 120 Cal Fat: 0 g Carbohydrates: 1 g Protein: 6 g Fiber: 2 g

420. *Sprouts and Apple Snack Salad*

Preparation Time: 10 minutes - **Cooking Time:** 0 minute - **Servings:** 4

- 1-pound brussels sprouts, shredded
- 1 cup walnuts, chopped
- 1 apple, cored and cubed
- 1 red onion, chopped

For the salad dressing:

- 3 tablespoons red vinegar
- 1 tablespoon mustard
- 1/2 cup olive oil
- 1 garlic clove, minced
- Black pepper to the taste

1. In a salad bowl, mix sprouts with apple, onion and walnuts.
2. In another bowl, mix vinegar with mustard, oil, garlic and pepper, whisk well, add this to your salad, toss well and serve as a snack.
Nutrition: Calories: 120 Cal Fat: 2 g Carbohydrates: 8 g Protein: 6 g Fiber: 2 g

421. *Celery and Raisins Snack Salad*

Preparation Time: 10 minutes - **Cooking Time:** 0 minutes - **Servings:** 4

- ½ cup raisins
- 4 cups celery, sliced
- ¼ cup parsley, chopped
- ½ cup walnuts, chopped
- Juice of ½ lemon

- 2 tablespoons olive oil
- Salt and black pepper to the taste

1. In a salad bowl.
2. Mix celery with raisins, walnuts, parsley, lemon juice, oil and black pepper, toss
3. Divide into small cups and serve as a snack.
Nutrition: Calories: 120 Cal Fat: 1 g Carbohydrates: 6 g Protein: 5 g Fiber: 2 g

422. Mozzarella Bars

Preparation Time: 10 minutes - **Cooking Time:** 40 minutes - **Servings:** 12
- 1 big cauliflower head, riced
- ½ cup low-fat mozzarella cheese, shredded
- ¼ cup egg whites
- 1 teaspoon Italian seasoning
- Black pepper to the taste

1. Spread the cauliflower rice on a lined baking sheet, cook in the oven at 375 degrees F for 20 minutes.
2. Transfer to a bowl, add black pepper, cheese, seasoning and egg whites.
3. Stir well, spread into a rectangle pan and press on the bottom.
4. Introduce in the oven at 375 degrees F, bake for 20 minutes, cut into 12 bars.
5. and serve as a snack.
Nutrition: Calories: 140 Cal Fat: 1 g Carbohydrates: 6 g Protein: 6 g Fiber: 3 g

423. Eggplant Salsa

Preparation Time: 10 minutes - **Cooking Time:** 10 minutes - **Servings:** 4
- 1 AND ½ CUPS TOMATOES, CHOPPED
- 3 cups eggplant, cubed
- a drizzle of olive oil
- 2 teaspoons capers
- 6 ounces green olives, pitted and sliced
- 4 garlic cloves, minced
- 2 teaspoons balsamic vinegar
- 1 tablespoon basil, chopped
- black pepper to the taste

1. Heat a pan with the oil over medium-high heat, add eggplant, stirand cook for 5 minutes. Add tomatoes, capers, olives, garlic, vinegar, basil and black pepper, toss, cook for 5 minutes more, divide into small cupsand serve cold.
Nutrition: Calories: 120 Cal Fat: 6 g Carbohydrates: 9 g Protein: 7 g Fiber: 5 g

424. Date Nut Bread

Preparation Time: 30 minutes - **Cooking Time:** 4-6 hours - **Servings:** 4-6
- ¾ cup Medjool dates
- 1 ¼ cup All-Purpose flour
- 2 teaspoon baking powder
- ¼ teaspoon baking soda
- ½ teaspoon salt
- ½ cup sugar
- ¾ cup milk
- 1 egg, slightly beaten
- 1 tablespoon orange peel, grated
- 1 tablespoon coconut oil, melted
- ¼ cup buckwheat flour
- 1 cup walnuts, chopped

1. On a chopping board, put the dates and sprinkle 1 tablespoon of All-Purpose flour over them. Dip a knife into the flour and finely chop the dates. Flour the knife sometimes to avoid sticking the cut-up fruit together.
2. Sift the remaining All-Purpose flour, baking powder, baking soda, salt and sugar into a large bowl.
3. Combine the milk, egg, orange peel and oil in a separate dish.
4. Add the buckwheat flour to the flour mixture, mix well and gently fold in the dates, along with any flour left on the cutting block and the walnuts.
5. Pour in the liquid **ingredients** and mix until just combined.
6. Transfer dough into a well-greased and floured baking unit. Cover and place in the slow cooker
7. Use a toothpick or small amount of twisted aluminum foil to prop the crockpot lid open a tiny fraction to allow steam to escape.
8. Cook on high for 4 to 6 hours. Cool on a rack for 10 minutes. Serve warm or cold.
9. Do NOT lift the crockpot lid while the bread is baking.
Nutrition: Calories: 70 Cal Fat:1 g Carbohydrates: 15 g Protein: 1 g Fiber: 1 g

425. Strawberry Rhubarb Crisp

Preparation Time: 10 minutes - **Cooking Time:** 45 minutes - **Servings:** 6-8
- 1 cup white sugar
- ½ cup buckwheat flour + 3 tablespoons
- 3 cups strawberries, sliced
- 3 cups rhubarb, diced
- ½ lemon, juiced
- 1 cup packed brown sugar
- 1 cup coconut oil, melted
- ¾ cup rolled oats
- ¼ cup buckwheat groats
- ¼ cup walnuts, chopped

1. Preheat oven to 375 degrees F
2. Combine the white sugar, 3 tablespoons of flour, strawberries, rhubarb, and lemon juice in a large bowl. Place a 9x13 inch baking dish with the mixture.
3. Mix ½ cup of flour, brown sugar, coconut oil, oats, buckwheat grits and walnuts in a separate bowl until crumbly. For this, you may wish to use a pastry blender. Crumble the rhubarb and strawberry mixture on top.
4. Bake in a preheated oven for 45 minutes, or until crisp and lightly browned.
Nutrition: Calories: 240 Cal Fat: 7 g Carbohydrates: 42 g Protein: 2 g Fiber: 3 g

426. Veggie Cakes

Preparation Time: 30 Minutes - **Cooking Time:** 30 Minutes - **Servings:** 8
- Two teaspoons ginger, grated
- 1 cup yellow onion, chopped
- 1 cup mushrooms, minced
- 1 cup canned red lentils, drained
- ¼ cup veggie stock
- One sweet potato, chopped
- ¼ cup parsley, chopped
- ¼ cup hemp seeds
- One tablespoon curry powder
- ¼ cup cilantro, chopped
- A drizzle of olive oil

- 1 cup quick oats
- Two tablespoons rice flour

1. Warmth a pan with the oil on medium-high heat, add ginger, onion, and mushrooms, stir, and cook for 2-3 minutes.
2. Add lentils, potato, and stock, stir, cook for 5-6 minutes, take off heat, cool the whole mixture, and mash it with a fork.
3. Add parsley, cilantro, hemp, oats, curry powder, and rice flour, stir well and shape medium cakes out of this mix.
4. Place veggie cakes in your air fryer's basket and cook at 3750 F for 10 minutes, flipping them halfway.
5. Serve them as an appetizer.
NUTRITION: Calories: 212 Fat: 4 grams Net Carbs: 8 grams Protein: 10 grams

427. *Cinnamon Coconut Chips*
Preparation Time: 7 Minutes - **Cooking Time:** 25 Minutes - **Servings:** 2
- ¼ cup coconut chips, unsweetened
- ¼ teaspoon of sea salt
- ¼ cup cinnamon

1. Add cinnamon and salt in a mixing bowl and set aside. Heat a pan over medium heat for 2 minutes.
2. Place the coconut chips in the hot pan and stir until coconut chips crisp and lightly brown.
3. Toss toasted coconut chips with cinnamon and salt.
NUTRITION: Calories: 228 Fat: 21 grams Net Carbs: 7.8 grams Protein: 1.9 grams

428. *Peach Cobbler*
Preparation Time: 20 Minutes - **Cooking Time:** 4 hours - **Servings:** 4
- 4 cups peaches, peeled and sliced
- ¼ cup of coconut sugar
- ½ teaspoon cinnamon powder
- 1 ½ cups vegan sweet crackers, crushed ¼ cup stevia
- ¼ teaspoon nutmeg, ground
- ½ cup almond milk
- One teaspoon vanilla extract
- Cooking spray

1. In a bowl, mix peaches with coconut sugar and cinnamon and stir.
2. In a separate bowl, mix crackers with stevia, nutmeg, almond milk, and vanilla extract and stir.
3. Shower your slow cooker with cooking spray and spread peaches on the bottom.
4. Add crackers mix, spread, cover, and cook on Low for 4 hours.
5. Divide cobbler between plates and serve.
NUTRITION: Calories: 212 Fat: 4 grams Net Carbs: 7 grams Protein: 3 grams

429. *Chocolate Brownies*
Preparation Time: 10 Minutes - **Cooking Time:** 20 Minutes - **Servings:** 4
- Two tablespoons cocoa powder
- One scoop protein powder
- 1 cup bananas, over-ripe
- ½ cup almond butter, melted

1. Preheat the oven to 3500 F.
2. Spray the brownie pan with cooking spray.
3. Add the real ingredients in your blender and blend until smooth.

4. Pour the batter into the prepared pan.
5. Put in the oven for 20 minutes.
NUTRITION: Calories: 82 Fat: 2.1 grams Net Carbs: 11.4 grams Protein:6.9 grams

430. *The Keto Lovers "Magical" Grain-Free Granola*
Preparation Time: 30 Minutes - **Cooking Time:** 1 Hour and 15 Minutes - **Servings:**
- ½ cup of raw sunflower seeds
- ½ cup of raw hemp hearts
- ½ cup of flaxseeds
- ¼ cup of chia seeds
- Two tablespoons of Psyllium Husk powder
- One tablespoon of cinnamon
- Stevia
- ½ teaspoon of baking powder
- ½ teaspoon of salt
- 1 cup of water

1. Preheat your oven to 3000 F. Make sure to line a baking page with a parchment piece.
2. Take your food processor and grind all the seeds.
3. Add the dry ingredients and mix well.
4. Stir in water until fully incorporated.
5. Let the mixture sit for a while. Wait until it thickens up.
6. Spread the mixture evenly-giving a thickness of about ¼ inch.
7. Bake for 45 minutes.
8. Break apart the granola and keep baking for another 30 minutes until the pieces are crunchy.
9. Remove and allow them to cool.
NUTRITION: Calories: 292 Fat: 25 grams Net Carbs: 12 grams Protein: 8 grams

431. *Keto Ice Cream*
Preparation Time: 10 Minutes - **Cooking Time:** 3-4 Hours to Freeze - **Servings:** 4-5
- 1 ½ teaspoon of natural vanilla extract
- 1/8 teaspoon of salt
- 1/3 cup of erythritol
- 2 cups of artificial coconut milk, full fat

1. Stir together the vanilla extract, salt, sweetener, and milk.
2. If you do not come up with an ice cream machine, freeze the mixture in ice cube trays, then use a high-speed blender to blend the frozen cubes or thaw them enough to meld in a regular blender or food processor.
3. If you have an ice cream machine, just blend according to the manufacturer's directions.
4. Eat as it is or freeze for a firmer texture.
NUTRITION: Calories: 184 Fat: 19.1 grams Net Carbs: 4.4 grams Protein: 1.8 grams

432. *Apple Mix*
Preparation Time: 10 Minutes - **Cooking Time:** 4 Hours - **Servings:** 6
- Six apples, cored, peeled, and sliced
- 1½ cups almond flour
- Cooking spray
- 1 cup of coconut sugar
- One tablespoon cinnamon powder
- ¾ cup cashew butter, melted

1. Add apple slices to your slow cooker after you have greased it with cooking spray.
2. Add flour, sugar, cinnamon, and coconut butter, stir gently, cover, cook on High for 4 hours, divide into bowls and serve cold.
NUTRITION: Calories: 200 Fat: 5 grams Net Carbs: 8 grams Protein: 4 grams

433. Almond Butter Fudge
Preparation Time: 17 Minutes - **Cooking Time:** 2-3 Hours to Freeze - **Servings:** 8
- 2 ½ tablespoons coconut oil
- 2 ½ tablespoons honey
- ½ cup almond butter

1. In a saucepan, pour almond butter then add coconut oil warm for 2 minutes or until melted.
2. Add honey and stir.
3. Pour the mixture into a candy container and store it in the fridge until set.
NUTRITION: Calories: 63 Fat: 4.8 grams Net Carbs: 5.6 grams Protein: 0.2 grams

434. The Vegan Pumpkin Spicy Fat Bombs
Preparation Time: 20 Minutes - **Cooking Time:** 1 Hour and 20 Minutes - **Servings:** 12
- ¾ cup of pumpkin puree
- ¼ cup of hemp seeds
- ½ cup of coconut oil
- Two teaspoons of pumpkin pie spice
- One teaspoon of vanilla extract
- Liquid Stevia

1. Take a blender and add together all the ingredients.
2. Blend them well and portion the mixture out into silicon molds.
3. Allow them to chill and enjoy!
NUTRITION: Calories: 103 Fat: 10 grams Net Carbs: 2 grams Protein: 1 gram

435 Orange Cake
Preparation Time: 25 Minutes - **Cooking Time:** 5 Hours and 10 Minutes - **Servings:** 4
- Cooking spray
- One teaspoon baking powder
- 1 cup almond flour
- 1 cup of coconut sugar
- ½ teaspoon cinnamon powder
- Three tablespoons coconut oil, melted
- ½ cup almond milk
- ½ cup pecans, chopped
- ¾ cup of water
- ½ cup raisins
- ½ cup orange peel, grated
- ¾ cup of orange juice

1. In a bowl, mix flour with half of the sugar, baking powder, cinnamon, two tablespoons oil, milk, pecans, and raisins, stir and pour this in your slow cooker after you have sprayed it with cooking spray.
2. Warm a small pan over medium heat. Add water, orange juice, orange peel, the rest of the oil, and the remainder of the sugar, stir, bring to a boil, pour over the blend in the slow cooker, cover, and cook on Low for 5 hours.
3. Divide into dessert bowls and serve cold.

NUTRITION: Calories: 182 Fat: 3 grams Net Carbs: 4 grams Protein: 3 grams

436. Chia Raspberry Pudding
Preparation Time: 10 Minutes - **Cooking Time:** 3 Hours - **Servings:** 2
Four tablespoons chia seeds
- ½ cup raspberries
- 1 cup of coconut milk

1. Add the raspberry and coconut milk into your blender and blend until smooth.
2. Pour the mixture into a mason jar.
3. Add chia seeds and stir.
4. Cap jar and shake.
5. Set in the fridge for 3 hours.
NUTRITION: Calories: 408 Fat: 38.8 grams Net Carbs: 22.3 grams Protein: 9.1 grams

437. Pumpkin Cake
Preparation Time: 20 Minutes - **Cooking Time:** 2 Hours and 10 Minutes - **Servings:** 10
- 1 ½ teaspoons baking powder
- Cooking spray
- 1 cup pumpkin puree
- 2 cups almond flour
- ½ teaspoon baking soda
- 1 ½ teaspoons cinnamon, ground
- ¼ teaspoon ginger, ground
- One tablespoon coconut oil, melted
- One tablespoon flaxseed mixed with two tablespoons water
- One tablespoon vanilla extract
- 1/3 cup maple syrup
- One teaspoon lemon juice

1. In a bowl, flour with baking powder, baking soda, cinnamon, and ginger, then stir.
2. Add flaxseed, coconut oil, and vanilla, pumpkin puree, and maple syrup, and lemon juice, stir and pour in your slow cooker after spraying it with cooking spray parchment paper.
3. Cover Up pot and cook on Low for 2 hours and 20 minutes.
4. Leave the cake to cool down, slice, and serve.
NUTRITION: Calories: 182 Fat: 3 grams Net Carbs: 3 grams Protein: 1 gram

438. Apple Crisp
Preparation Time: 10 Minutes - **Cooking Time:** 40 Minutes - **Servings:** 6
- ½ cup vegan butter
- Six large apples, diced large
- 1 cup dried cranberries
- Two tablespoons granulated sugar
- Two teaspoons ground cinnamon, divided
- ¼ teaspoon ground nutmeg
- ¼ teaspoon ground ginger
- Two teaspoons lemon juice
- 1 cup all-purpose flour
- 1 cup rolled oats
- 1 cup brown sugar
- ¼ teaspoon salt

1. Preheat the oven to 350°F. Gently grease an 8-inch square baking dish with butter or cooking spray.

2. Make the filling. Combine the apples, cranberries, granulated sugar, a teaspoon of cinnamon, nutmeg, ginger and lemon juice in a large bowl. Toss to coat. Move the apple mixture to the prepared baking dish.

3. Make the topping. In the same large bowl, now empty, combine the all-purpose flour, oats, brown sugar, and salt. Stir to combine. Add Up the butter and, using a pastry cutter (or two knives moving in a crisscross pattern), cut back the butter into the flour and oat mixture until the butter is small.

4. Spread the topping over the apples evenly, patting down slightly— Bake for 35 minutes or until golden and bubbly.

NUTRITION: Calories: 488 Total Fat: 9 G Carbs: 101 G Fiber: 10 G Protein: 5 G Calcium: 50 Mg Vitamin D: 0 Mcg Vitamin B12: 0 Mcg Iron: 2 Mg Zinc: 1 Mg

439. *Secret Ingredient Chocolate Brownies*

Preparation Time: 10 Minutes - **Cooking Time:** 35 Minutes - **Servings:** 6 to 8

- ¾ cup flour
- ¼ teaspoon baking soda
- ¼ teaspoon salt
- ⅓ Cup vegan butter
- ¾ cup of sugar
- Two tablespoon water
- 1¼ cups semi-sweet or dark dairy-free chocolate chips
- Six tablespoons aquafaba, divided
- One teaspoon vanilla extract

1. Preheat the oven to 325°F. Line Up a 9-inch square baking pan with parchment or grease well.

2. In a large bowl, combine the flour, baking soda, and salt. Set aside.

3. In a medium saucepan, mix up the butter, sugar, and water. Bring to a boil, stirring occasionally. Reduce from heat and stir in the chocolate chips.

4. Whisk in 3 tablespoons of aquafaba until thoroughly combined. Add the vanilla extract and the remaining three tablespoons of aquafaba, and whisk until mixed.

5. Apply the mixture of chocolate to the mixture of flour and whisk until it is combined. Into the prepared tub, pour down in an even layer. Bake till the top is set for 35 minutes, but when slightly shaken, the brownie jiggles. Enable 45 minutes to 1 hour to cool completely, before removing and serving.

NUTRITION: Calories: 369 Total Fat: 19 G Carbs: 48 G Fiber: 1 G Protein:4 G Calcium: 1 Mg Vitamin D: 0 Mcg Vitamin B12: 0 Mcg Iron: 1 Mg Zinc:0 Mg

440. *Chocolate Chip Pecan Cookies*

Preparation Time: 10 Minutes - **Cooking Time:** 16 Minutes - **Servings:** 30 Small Cookies

- ¾ cup pecan halves, toasted
- 1 cup vegan butter
- ½ teaspoon salt
- ½ cup powdered sugar
- Two teaspoons vanilla extract
- 2 cups all-purpose flour
- 1 cup mini dairy-free chocolate chips

1. Preheat the oven to 350°F. Line a large rimmed baking page with parchment paper.

2. In a small skillet over medium heat, toast the pecans until warm and fragrant, about 2 minutes. Remove from the pan. Once these are cool, chop them into small pieces.

3. Make use of an electric hand mixer or a stand mixer fitted with a paddle attachment, combine the butter, salt, and powdered sugar, and cream together on high speed for 3 to 4 minutes, until light and fluffy. Stir in the vanilla extract, then beat for 1 minute or so. Turn the mixer on low and slowly add the flour, ½ cup at a time, until a dough form. Combine the chocolate chips and pecans and mix until just incorporated.

4. Using your hands, a large spoon, or a 1-inch ice cream scoop, drop 1-inch balls of dough on the baking sheet, spread out 1 inch apart. Gently press down on the cookies to flatten them slightly. Bake for 10 to 15 minutes. Wait until just yellow around the edges. Let it cool for 5 minutes.

5. Transfer them to a wire rack. Serve or store in an airtight container.

NUTRITION: Calories: 152 Total Fat: 11 G Carbs: 13 G Fiber: 1 G Protein:2 G Calcium: 2 Mg Vitamin D: 0 Mcg Vitamin B12: 0 Mcg Iron: 0 Mg Zinc:0 Mg

441. *No-Bake Chocolate Coconut Energy Balls*

Period of Preparation: 15 Minutes - **Cooking Time:** 3 to 4 Chilling Hours - **Servings:** 9 Energy Balls

- ¼ cup dry roasted or raw pumpkin seeds ¼ cup dry roasted or raw sunflower seeds ½ cup unsweetened shredded coconut Two tablespoons chia seeds ¼ teaspoon salt
- 1½ tablespoons Dutch-process cocoa powder ¼ cup rolled oats
- Two tablespoons coconut oil, melted
- Six pitted dates
- Two tablespoons all-natural almond butter

1. Mix the pumpkin seeds, sunflower seeds, coconut, chia seeds, salt, cocoa powder, and oats in a food processor. Pulse until the mix is coarsely crumbled.

2. Add the coconut oil, dates, and almond butter. Pulse until the mixture is fused and sticks together when squeezed between your fingers.

3. Scoop out two tablespoons of the mix at a time and roll them into 1½-inch balls with your hands. Place them spaced apart on a freezer-safe plate and freeze for 15 minutes. Remove from the freezer and keep refrigerated in an airtight container for up to 4 days.

NUTRITION: Calories: 230 Total Fat: 12 G Carbs: 27 G Fiber: 5 G Protein:5 G

442. *Blueberry Hand Pies*

Preparation Time: 6 to 8 Minutes - **Cooking Time:** 20 Minutes plus Chill Time - **Servings:** 6 to 8

- 3 cups all-purpose flour, plus extra for sifting work surface ½ teaspoon salt
- ¼ cup, plus two tablespoons granulated sugar, divided
- 1 cup vegan butter
- ½ cup of cold water
- 1 cup fresh blueberries
- Two teaspoons lemon zest
- Two teaspoons lemon juice
- ¼ teaspoon ground cinnamon
- One teaspoon cornstarch
- ¼ cup unsweetened soy milk
- Coarse sugar, for sprinkling

1. Preheat the oven to 375°F. Set aside.

2. In a large bowl, merge the flour, salt, two tablespoons of granulated sugar, and vegan butter. Using a pastry cutter or two knives moving in a crisscross pattern, cut the butter into the other ingredients until the butter is small peas.

3. Add the cold water and knead to form a dough. Tear the dough in half and wrap the halves separately in plastic wrap. Refrigerate for 15 minutes.

4. Make the blueberry filling. In a medium bowl, mix the blueberries, lemon zest, lemon juice, cinnamon, cornstarch, and the remaining ¼ cup of sugar.

5. Remove one half of the dough. On a floured side, roll out the dough to ¼- to ½-inch thickness. Turn a 5-inch bowl upside down, and, using it as a guide, cut the dough into circles to make mini pie crusts. Reroll scrap dough to cut out more circles. Repeat with the second half of the dough. You should come to an end up with 8 to 10 circles. Place the circles on the prepared sheet pan.

6. Spoon 1½ tablespoons of blueberry filling onto each circle, leaving a ¼-inch border and folding the circles in half to cover the filling, forming a half-moon shape. Use a fork to press the edges of the dough to seal the pies.

7. When all the pies are assembled, use a paring knife to score the pies by cutting three lines through the top crusts. Brush each pie with soy milk and sprinkle with coarse sugar. Bake for 20 minutes or until the filling is bubbly and the tops are golden. Let cool before serving.

NUTRITION: Calories: 416 Total Fat: 23 G Carbs: 46 G Fiber: 5 G Protein: 6 G

443. Date Squares

Preparation Time: 20 Minutes - **Cooking Time:** 25 Minutes - **Servings:** 12

- Cooking spray, for greasing
- 1½ cups rolled oats
- 1½ cups all-purpose flour
- ¾ cup, plus ⅓ cup brown sugar, divided
- ½ teaspoon ground cinnamon
- ¼ teaspoon ground nutmeg
- One teaspoon baking soda
- ¼ teaspoon salt
- ¾ cup vegan butter
- 18 pitted dates
- One teaspoon lemon zest
- One teaspoon lemon juice
- 1 cup of water

1. Preheat the oven to 350°F. Lightly grease or shower an 8-inch square baking plate. Set aside.

2. Make the base and topping mixture. In a large bowl, blend the rolled oats, flour, and ¾ cup of brown sugar, cinnamon, nutmeg, baking soda, and salt. Combine the butter and, using a pastry cutter or two knives working in a crisscross motion, cut the butter into the blend to form a crumbly dough. Press half of the dough into the prepared baking dish and set the remaining half aside.

3. To make a date filling, place a small saucepan over medium heat. Add the dates, the remaining ⅓ cup of sugar, the lemon zest, lemon juice, and water. Bring to a boil and cook for 7 to 10 minutes, until thickened.

4. When cooked, pour the date mixture over the dough base in the baking dish and top with the remaining crumb dough. Gently press down and spread evenly to cover all the filling. Bake for 25 minutes until lightly golden on top. Cool before serving. Store in an airtight container.

NUTRITION: Calories: 443 Total Fat: 12 G Carbs: 81 G Fiber: 7 G Protein:5 G

444. Homemade Chocolates with Coconut and Raisins

Preparation Time: 10 Minutes - **Cooking Time:** Chilling time - **Servings:** 20

- 1/2 cup cacao butter, melted
- 1/3 cup peanut butter
- 1/4 cup agave syrup
- A pinch of grated nutmeg
- A pinch of coarse salt
- 1/2 teaspoon vanilla extract
- 1 cup dried coconut, shredded
- 6 ounces dark chocolate, chopped
- 3 ounces raisins

1. Carefully combine all the ingredients, not including for the chocolate, in a mixing bowl.

2. Spoon the mixture into molds. Leave to set hard in a cool place.

3. Melt the dark chocolate in your microwave. Pour in the melted chocolate until the fillings are covered. Leave to set hard in a cool place.

NUTRITION: Calories: 130 Fat: 9.1g Carbs: 12.1g Protein: 1.3g

445. Easy Mocha Fudge

Preparation Time: 10 Minutes - **Cooking Time:** 60 Minutes - **Servings:** 20

- 1 cup cookies, crushed
- 1/2 cup almond butter
- 1/4 cup agave nectar
- 6 ounces dark chocolate, broken into chunks
- One teaspoon instant coffee
- A pinch of grated nutmeg
- A pinch of salt

1. Line a large baking layer with parchment paper.

2. Melt the chocolate in your microwave and add in the remaining ingredients; stir to combine well.

3. Scrape the batter into a parchment-lined baking sheet. Put it in your freezer for a minimum of 1 hour to set.

4. Cut into squares and serve. Bon appétit!

NUTRITION: Calories: 105 Fat: 5.6g Carbs: 12.9g Protein: 1.1g

446. Almond and Chocolate Chip Bars

Preparation Time: 10 Minutes - **Cooking Time:** 30 Minutes - **Servings:** 10

- 1/2 cup almond butter
- 1/4 cup coconut oil, melted
- 1/4 cup agave syrup
- One teaspoon vanilla extract
- 1/4 teaspoon sea salt
- 1/4 teaspoon grated nutmeg
- 1/2 teaspoon ground cinnamon
- 2 cups almond flour
- 1/4 cup flaxseed meal
- 1 cup vegan chocolate, cut into chunks
- 1 1/3 cups almonds, ground
- Two tablespoons cacao powder
- 1/4 cup agave syrup

1. In a mixing bowl, thoroughly combine the almond butter, coconut oil, 1/4 cup of agave syrup, vanilla, salt, nutmeg, and cinnamon.

2. Gradually stir in the almond flour and flaxseed meal and stir to combine. Add in the chocolate chunks and stir again.

3. In a small blending bowl, combine the almonds, cacao powder, and agave syrup. Now, spread the ganache onto the cake. Freeze for about 30 minutes, cut into bars and serve well chilled. Enjoy!

NUTRITION: Calories: 295 Fat: 17g Carbs: 35.2g Protein: 1.7g

447. Almond Butter Cookies

Preparation Time: 10 Minutes - **Cooking Time:** 30 Minutes - **Servings:** 10

- 3/4 cup all-purpose flour
- 1/2 teaspoon baking soda
- 1/4 teaspoon kosher salt
- One flax egg
- 1/4 cup coconut grease, at room temperature
- Two tablespoons almond milk
- 1/2 cup brown sugar
- 1/2 cup almond butter
- 1/2 teaspoon ground cinnamon
- 1/2 teaspoon vanilla

1. In a blending bowl, blend the flour, baking soda, and salt. In another bowl, combine the flax egg, coconut oil, almond milk, sugar, almond butter, cinnamon, and vanilla. Whisk the wet mixture into the dry materials and stir until well combined.

2. Place the batter in your refrigerator for about 30 minutes. Shape the batter into small cookies and arrange them on a parchment-lined cookie pan.

3. Bake in the preheated oven at 350 degrees F for approximately 12 minutes. Later, move the pan to a wire rack to cool at room temperature. Bon appétit!

NUTRITION: Calories: 197 Fat: 15.8g Carbs: 12.5g Protein: 2.1g

448. Vanilla Halvah Fudge

Preparation Time: 10 Minutes - **Cooking Time:** Chilling Time - **Servings:** 16

- 1/2 cup cocoa butter
- 1/2 cup tahini
- Eight dates pitted
- 1/4 teaspoon ground cloves
- A pinch of grated nutmeg
- A coarse pinch salt
- One teaspoon vanilla extract

1. Line a square baking pot with parchment paper.

2. Mix the materials until everything is well incorporated.

3. Scrape the batter into the parchment-lined pan. Place it until it is ready for serving, in the fridge. Healthy appetite!

NUTRITION: Calories: 106 Fat: 9.8g Carbs: 4.5g Protein: 1.4g

449. Raw Chocolate Mango Pie

Preparation Time: 10 Minutes - **Cooking Time:** Chilling Time - **Servings:** 16

- Avocado layer:
- Three ripe avocados, pitted and peeled
- A pinch of sea salt
- A pinch of ground anise
- 1/2 teaspoon vanilla paste
- Two tablespoons coconut milk

- Five tablespoons agave syrup
- 1/3 cup cocoa powder
- Crema layer:
- 1/3 cup almond butter
- 1/2 cup coconut cream
- One medium mango, peeled
- 1/2 coconut flakes
- Two tablespoons agave syrup

1. In your food processor, blend the avocado layer until smooth and uniform, reserve.

2. Then, blend the other layer in a separate bowl. Spoon the layers in a lightly oiled baking pan.

3. Transfer the cake to your freezer for about 3 hours. Store in your freezer. Bon appétit!

NUTRITION: Calories: 196 Fat: 16.8g Carbs: 14.1g Protein: 1.8g

450. Raw Raspberry Cheesecake

Preparation Time: 15 Minutes - **Cooking Time:** Chilling Time - **Servings:** 9

Crust:
- 2 cups almonds
- 1 cup fresh dates, pitted
- 1/4 teaspoon ground cinnamon

Filling:
- 2 cups raw cashews, drenched overnight and drained
- 14 ounces blackberries, frozen
- One tablespoon fresh lime juice
- 1/4 teaspoon crystallized ginger
- One can use coconut cream
- Eight fresh dates pitted

1. In your food processor, blend the crust ingredients until the mixture comes together; press the crust into a lightly oiled springform pan.

2. Then, blend the filling layer until completely smooth. Spoon the filling onto the crust, creating a flat surface with a spatula. Transfer the cake to your freezer for about 3 hours. Store in your freezer. Garnish with organic citrus peel. Bon appétit!

NUTRITION: Calories: 385 Fat: 22.9 Carbs: 41.1g Protein: 10.8g

Beverage

451. Matcha Green Juice

Preparation time: 10 minutes - **Cooking time:** 0 minutes - **Total time:** 10 minutes - **Servings:** 2

- 5 ounces fresh kale
- 2 ounces fresh arugula
- ¼ cup fresh parsley
- 4 celery stalks
- 1 green apple, cored and chopped
- 1 (1-inch) piece fresh ginger, peeled
- 1 lemon, peeled
- ½ teaspoon matcha green tea

1. Add all ingredients into a juicer and extract the juice according to the manufacturer's method.

2. Pour into 2 glasses and serve immediately.

Nutrition: Calories: 113 Sodium: 22 mg Dietary Fiber: 1.2 g Total Fat: 2.1 g Total Carbs: 12.3 g Protein: 1.3 g

452. Celery Juice

Preparation time: 10 minutes - Cooking time: 0 minutes -Servings: 2

- 8 celery stalks with leaves
- 2 tablespoons fresh ginger, peeled
- 1 lemon, peeled
- ½ cup filtered water
- Pinch of salt

1. In a mixer, put all the ingredients and pulse until well mixed.
2. Strain the juice and pass it into 2 glasses via a fine mesh strainer.
3. Serve immediately.

Nutrition: Calories: 32 Sodium: 21 mg Dietary Fiber: 1.4 g Total Fat: 1.1 g Total Carbs: 1.3 g Protein: 1.2 g

453. Kale & Orange Juice

Preparation time: 10 minutes - Cooking time: 0 minutes - Servings: 2

- 5 large oranges, peeled
- 2 bunches fresh kale

1. Add all ingredients into a juicer and extract the juice according to the manufacturer's method.
2. Pour into 2 glasses and serve immediately.

Nutrition: Calories: 315 Sodium: 34 mg Dietary Fiber: 1.3 g Total Fat: 4.1 g Total Carbs: 14.3 g Protein: 1.2 g

454. Apple & Cucumber Juice

Preparation time: 10 minutes - Cooking time: 0 minutes - Servings: 2

- 3 large apples, cored and sliced
- 2 large cucumbers, sliced
- 4 celery stalks
- 1 (1-inch) piece fresh ginger, peeled
- 1 lemon, peeled

1. Add all ingredients into a juicer and extract the juice according to the manufacturer's method.
2. Pour into 2 glasses and serve immediately.

Nutrition: Calories: 230 Sodium: 31 mg Dietary Fiber: 1.3 g Total Fat: 2.1 g Total Carbs: 1.3 g Protein: 1.2 g

455. Lemony Green Juice

Preparation time: 10 minutes - Cooking time: 0 minutes - Servings: 2

- 2 large green apples, cored and sliced
- 4 cups fresh kale leaves
- 4 tablespoons fresh parsley leaves
- 1 tablespoon fresh ginger, peeled
- 1 lemon, peeled
- ½ cup filtered water
- Pinch of salt

1. In a mixer, put all the ingredients and pulse until well mixed.
2. Via a fine mesh strainer, drain the juice and transfer it into 2 jars.
3. Serve immediately.

Nutrition: Calories: 196 Sodium: 21 mg Dietary Fiber: 1.4 g Total Fat: 1.1 g Total Carbs: 1.6 g Protein: 1.5 g

456. Creamy Strawberry & Cherry Smoothie

Preparation Time: 10 minutes - Cooking Time: 15 minutes - Servings: 1

- 3½ ounces of strawberries
- 3.5 ounces of frozen pitted cherries
- 1 tablespoon plain full-fat yogurt
- 6.5 ounces of unsweetened soya milk

1. Place the ingredients into a blender, then process until smooth.

Nutrition: Calories: 203 Sodium: 23 mg Dietary Fiber: 1.4 g Total Fat: 3.1 g Total Carbs: 12.3 g Protein: 1.7 g

457. Matcha Green Tea Smoothie

Preparation Time: 3 minutes - Cooking time: 0 minute - Serves: 2

- 2 ripe bananas 2
- 2 teaspoons matcha green tea powder
- 2 teaspoons honey
- 1/2 teaspoon vanilla bean paste (not extract) or a small scrape of
- the seeds from a vanilla pod
- 250 ml of milk
- Six ice cubes

1. Blend all the ingredients in a mixer and serve in two glasses.

Nutrition: Calories: 183 Sodium: 26 mg Dietary Fiber: 1.4 g Total Fat: 2.1 g Total Carbs: 12.1 g Protein: 1.2 g

458. Green Tea Smoothie

Preparation time: 10 minutes - Cooking time: 0 minutes - Servings: 1

- 1 ripe large banana
- Milk
- ¼ teaspoon vanilla bean paste
- 3 ice cubes
- 1 teaspoon honey

1. In a mixer, blend all the ingredients together and serve in a glass.

Nutrition: Calories: 185 Sodium: 21 mg Dietary Fiber: 1.3 g Total Fat: 2.1 g Total Carbs: 10.3 g Protein: 1.2 g

459. Chocolate Balls

Preparation Time: 10 minutes - Cooking Time: 15 minutes - Servings: 1

- 2 ounces of peanut butter or almond butter
- 1 ounce of cocoa powder
- 1 ounce of desiccated shredded coconut
- 1 tablespoon honey
- 1 tablespoon cocoa powder for coating

1. Mix all ingredients into a bowl. Scoop out a little of the mixture and shape it into a ball.
2. Roll the ball in a little cocoa powder and set aside
3. Repeat for the remaining mixture. It can be consumed immediately or kept in the fridge.

Nutrition: Calories: 295 Sodium: 24 mg Dietary Fiber: 1.4 g Total Fat: 4.1 g Total Carbs: 16.3 g Protein: 1.3 g

460. Strawberry & Citrus Blend

Preparation Time: 10 minutes - Cooking Time: 15 minutes - Servings: 1

- 3 ounces of strawberries
- 1 apple, cored
- 1 orange, peeled
- ½ avocado, peeled and de-stoned
- ½ teaspoon matcha powder
- Juice of 1 lime

1. Place ingredients into a blender with enough water to cover them and process until smooth.

Nutrition: Calories: 124 Sodium: 31 mg Dietary Fiber: 1.4 g Total Fat: 2.1 g Total Carbs: 12.2 g Protein: 1.2 g

461. Turmeric Tea

Preparation time: 10 minutes - Servings: 1
- 1 ½ heaped teaspoon turmeric powder
- ½ tablespoon fresh ginger, grated
- 1 small lemon
- Orange zest
- 1 teaspoon honey.

1. Boil 200ml of water in the kettle
2. In a teapot or jug, place the turmeric, ginger, and orange zest. Pour the boiling water over and quit to stand for 5 minutes.
3. Strain into a cup through a sieve or tea strainer, add lemon juice or a lemon slice and sweeten with honey.

Nutrition: Calories: 83 Sodium: 21 mg Dietary Fiber: 1.4 g Total Fat: 1.1 g Total Carbs: 1.3 g Protein: 1.2 g

462. Strawberry and Blackcurrant Jelly

Preparation time: 10 minutes - Cooking time: 0 minute - Servings: 2
- Strawberries, hulled and chopped Blackcurrants washed and stalks removed
- Water
- 3 tablespoons granulated sugar.
- 4 gelatin leaves

1. Arrange the strawberries in 4 serving dishes.
2. To soften the gelatin leaves, place them in a bowl of cold water.
3. In a small pan with sugar and 200ml of water, put the blackcurrants and simmer. For 5 minutes, boil vigorously and then remove from the flame. Leave for 2 minutes to stand
4. Squeeze out the gelatin leaves with extra water and apply them to the blackcurrant mixture. Stir until it is fully dissolved, then stir in the remaining water.
5. Pour the liquid into the dishes that are prepared and refrigerate until set.The jelly should be ready in about 3 to 4 hours or you can leave it overnight.

Nutrition: Calories: 232 Sodium: 24 mg Dietary Fiber: 1.4 g Total Fat: 2.1 g Total Carbs: 10.3 g Protein: 1.2 g

463. Green Juice Salad

Preparation time: 10 minutes - Cooking time: 0 minute - Servings: 1
- 2 handfuls of chopped kale
- 1 handful of chopped arugulas
- 1 tablespoon chopped parsley
- 2 stalks of celery, sliced into bite-sized pieces ½ green apple, chopped into bite-sized pieces 6 walnuts, crushed
- 1 tablespoon olive oil
- ½ lemon, juiced
- 1 teaspoon grated ginger

- A pinch of salt and pepper

1. To complete this recipe, you will need to do the following:
2. Mix the juice of the lemon, ginger, seasonings, and olive oil into a small jar or small Tupperware container. Put it aside until it's ready to feed.
3. Add your kale, arugula, parsley, celery, apple, and walnut to a big bowl or large Tupperware jar. When you are ready to eat, mix it up until well mixed and set aside.
4. Shake up the dressing until you are ready to eat it, then apply it to the bowl and mix it thoroughly.

Nutrition: Calories: 385 Sodium: 32 mg Dietary Fiber: 1.2 g Total Fat: 4.1 g Total Carbs: 12.3 g Protein: 1.3 g

464. Sirtfood Smoothie

Preparation time: 10 minutes - Cooking time: 0 minutes - Servings: 2
- 3 ounces of plain Greek yogurt (or vegan alternative, such as soy or coconut yogurt)
- 6 walnut halves
- 10 medium strawberries, hulled
- A handful of kale stalks removed
- 1 ounce of dark chocolate (85 percent cocoa solids)
- 1 Medjool date, pitted
- 1/2 teaspoon ground turmeric
- 1 small size chili
- 7/8 cup (200ml) unsweetened almond milk.
- 1 teaspoon honey

1. Blend all the ingredients in a blender until smooth and serve in a glass.

Nutrition: Calories: 162, Sodium: 28 mg, Dietary Fiber: 1.4 g, Total Fat: 3.1 g, Total Carbs: 11.3 g, Protein: 1.2 g.

465. Centrifuged Green Juice

Preparation time: 10 minutes - Cooking time: 0 minutes - Servings: 2
- 1.3 ounce of kale
- 1.5 ounce of rocket salad
- 0.7 ounce of parsley
- 5 ounces of green celery with the leaves
- 1/2 green apple
- 1/2 lemon juice
- 1/2 teaspoon of matcha tea

1. Centrifuge the kale, rocket salad and parsley; add grated celery and apple; enrich with half a squeezed lemon and half a teaspoon of matcha tea.
2. Drink immediately so as not to lose the beneficial effects of vegetables and not keep it in the fridge. It should always be prepared when consuming it.

Nutrition: Calories: 150 Sodium: 32 mg Dietary Fiber: 1.4 g Total Fat: 2.1 g Total Carbs: 7.3 g Protein: 1.2 g

466. Iced Cranberry Green Juice

Preparation time: 10 minutes - Cooking time: 30 minutes - Servings: 1
- 5fl Oz light cranberry juice
- 3½fl Oz green tea, cooled
- Squeeze of lemon juice
- A handful of crushed ice (optional)
- Sprig of mint

1. Pour the green tea and cranberry into a glass and add a squeeze of lemon juice.
2. Top it off with some ice and garnish with a mint leaf.

Nutrition: Calories: 14 Sodium: 23 mg Dietary Fiber: 1.4 g Total Fat: 2.1 g Total Carbs: 1.3 g Protein: 1.2 g

467. Ginger & Turmeric Juice

Preparation time: 10 minutes - Cooking time: 7 minutes - Servings: 1
- 1-inch chunk fresh ginger root, peeled
- ¼ teaspoon turmeric
- 1 teaspoon of honey (optional)
- Ice

1. Make incisions in the piece of root ginger, without cutting all the way through.
2. Place the ginger and turmeric in a cup and pour in boiling water. Allow it to steep for 7 minutes.
3. Apply a teaspoon of honey if you wish. Let it cook and then add ice and enjoy it.

Nutrition: Calories: 33 Sodium: 22 mg Dietary Fiber: 1.6 g Total Fat: 1.1g Total Carbs: 1.3 g Protein: 1.2 g

468. Orange & Kale Juice

Preparation Time: 10 minutes - **Servings: 2**
- 5 oranges, peeled 2 cups fresh kale

Add all ingredients into a juicer and extract the juice according to the manufacturer's method.
In case you don't have one, add all the ingredients in a blender and pulse until well combined.
Filter the juice and pass it into two glasses via a fine mesh strainer.

Nutrition Facts: Calories 52 kcal, Fat 0.7 g, Carbohydrate 8.5 g, Protein 1.5 g

469. Spinach Smoothie

Preparation Time: 5 minutes - **Servings: 1**
- 1 cup spinach
- 1 pear
- ½ bananas ¼ zucchini
- ½ cup almond milk, unsweetened

Add all ingredients in a high-power blender and pulse until smooth. Pour the smoothie into two glasses and serve immediately.

Nutrition Facts: Calories 123kcal, Fat 0.9 g, Carbohydrate 18.5 g, Protein 2.4 g

• 470. Lemony Apple & Kale Juice

Preparation Time: 10 minutes - **Servings: 2**
- 2 green apples, cored and sliced 4 cups fresh kale leaves
- 4 tbsp. fresh parsley leaves 1 tbsp. fresh ginger, peeled 1 lemon, peeled
- ½ cup filtered water Pinch of salt

Add all ingredients into a juicer and extract the juice according to the manufacturer's method.
In case you don't have one, add all the ingredients in a blender and pulse until well combined.
Filter the juice and pass it into two glasses via a fine mesh strainer. Serve immediately.

Nutrition Facts: Calories 55kcal, Fat 0.3 g, Carbohydrate 6.9 g, Protein 1.2 g

471. Apple & Celery Juice

Preparation Time: 10 minutes - **Servings: 2**

- 4 large green apples, cored and sliced 4 large celery stalks
- 1 lemon, peeled

Add all ingredients into a juicer and extract the juice according to the manufacturer's method.
In case you don't have one, add all the ingredients in a blender and pulse until well combined. Filter the juice and pass it into two glasses via a fine mesh strainer.. Serve immediately.

Nutrition Facts: Calories 62kcal, Fat 0.6 g, Carbohydrate 6.7 g, Protein 1.8 g

472. Apple, Orange & Broccoli Juice

Preparation Time: 10 minutes - **Servings: 2**
- 2 broccoli stalks, chopped
- 2 large green apples, cored and sliced 3 oranges, peeled - 4 tbsp. fresh parsley

Add all ingredients into a juicer and extract the juice according to the manufacturer's method.
In case you don't have one, add all the ingredients in a blender and pulse until well combined.
Filter the juice and pass it into two glasses via a fine mesh strainer.
Serve immediately.

Nutrition Facts: Calories 82kcal, Fat 0.3 g, Carbohydrate 8.5 g, Protein 2 g

473. Apple, Grapefruit & Carrot Juice

Preparation Time: 10 minutes - **Servings: 2**
- 3 cups fresh kale
- 2 large apples, cored and sliced
- 2 medium carrots, peeled and chopped
- 2 medium grapefruit, peeled and sectioned 1 tsp fresh lemon juice
- ½ cup filtered water

Add all ingredients into a juicer and extract the juice according to the manufacturer's method. In case you don't have one, add all the ingredients in a blender and pulse until well combined. Filter the juice and pass it into two glasses via a fine mesh strainer. Serve immediately.

Nutrition Facts: Calories 67kcal, Fat 0.2 g, Carbohydrate 8 g, Protein 0.8 g

474. Fruity Kale Juice

Preparation Time: 10 minutes - **Servings: 2**
- 2 large green apples, cored and sliced 2 large pears, cored and sliced
- 3 cups fresh kale leaves 3 celery stalks
- 1 lemon, peeled
- ½ cup filtered water

Add all ingredients into a juicer and extract the juice according to the manufacturer's method.
In case you don't have one, add all the ingredients in a blender and pulse until well combined.
Filter the juice and pass it into two glasses via a fine mesh strainer. Serve immediately.

Nutrition Facts: Calories 65kcal, Fat 0.3 g, Carbohydrate 5.9 g, Protein 2.5 g

475. Green Fruit Juice

Preparation Time: 10 minutes - **Servings: 2**
- 3 large kiwis, peeled and chopped

- 3 large green apples, cored and sliced 2 cups seedless green grapes
- 2 tsp fresh lime juice
- ½ cup filtered water

Add all ingredients into a juicer and extract the juice according to the manufacturer's method.

In case you don't have one, add all the ingredients in a blender and pulse until well combined.

Filter the juice and pass it into two glasses via a fine mesh strainer. Serve immediately.

Nutrition Facts: Calories 105kcal, Fat 0.5 g, Carbohydrate 12.5 g, Protein 1 g

476. Apple & Carrot Juice

Preparation Time: 10 minutes - **Servings:** 2
- 5 carrots, peeled and chopped
- 1 large apple, cored and chopped
- 1 ½-inch piece fresh ginger, peeled and chopped
- ½ of lemon
- ½ cup filtered water

Add all ingredients into a juicer and extract the juice according to the manufacturer's method.

In case you don't have one, add all the ingredients in a blender and pulse until well combined.

Filter the juice and pass it into two glasses via a fine mesh strainer. Serve immediately.

Nutrition Facts: Calories 125kcal, Fat 0.3 g, Carbohydrate 21.4 g Protein 1.7 g

477. Strawberry Juice

Preparation Time: 10 minutes - **Servings:** 2
- 2½ cups fresh ripe strawberries, hulled 1 apple, cored and chopped 1 lime, peeled

Add all ingredients into a juicer and extract the juice according to the manufacturer's method.

In case you don't have one, add all the ingredients in a blender and pulse until well combined.

Filter the juice and pass it into two glasses via a fine mesh strainer. Serve immediately. It can be stored in an acceptable container for up to 3 days in the refrigerator.

Nutrition Facts: Calories 108kcal, Fat 0.8 g, Carbohydrate 18.5 g, Protein 1.6 g

478. Chocolate and Date Smoothie

Preparation Time: 10 minutes - **Servings:** 2
- 4 Medjool dates, pitted 2 tbsp. cacao powder
- 2 tbsp. flaxseed
- 1 tbsp. almond butter 1 tsp vanilla extract ¼ tsp ground cinnamon
- 1½ cups almond milk, unsweetened 4 ice cubes

Add all ingredients in a high-power blender and pulse until smooth. Pour into two glasses and serve immediately.

It can be stored in an acceptable container for up to 3 days in the refrigerator.

Nutrition Facts: Calories 234kcal, Fat 5 g, Carbohydrate 25.5 g, Protein 6 g

479. Blueberry & Kale Smoothie

Preparation Time: 10 minutes - **Servings:** 2
- 2 cups frozen blueberries 2 cups fresh kale leaves 2 Medjool dates, pitted
- 1 tbsp. chia seeds

- 1 ½-inch piece fresh ginger, peeled and chopped 1½ cups almond milk, unsweetened

In a high-power blender, add all the ingredients and pulse until smooth. In two glasses, pour the smoothie and serve immediately.

It can be stored in an acceptable container for up to 3 days in the refrigerator.

Nutrition Facts: Calories 230kcal, Fat 4.5 g, Carbohydrate 28.8 g, Protein 5.6 g

480. Strawberry & Beet Smoothie

Preparation Time: 10 minutes - **Servings:** 2
- 2 cups frozen strawberries, pitted and chopped 2/3 cup frozen beets, chopped
- 1 ½-inch piece ginger, chopped
- 1 ½-inch piece fresh turmeric, chopped (or 1 tsp turmeric powder) ½ cup fresh orange juice
- 1 cup almond milk, unsweetened

Add all ingredients in a high-power blender and pulse until smooth. Pour the smoothie into two glasses and serve immediately.

It can be stored in an acceptable container for up to 3 days in the refrigerator.

Nutrition Facts: Calories 130kcal, Fat 0.2g, Carbohydrate 22.5 g, Protein 2 g

481. Green Pineapple Smoothie

Preparation Time: 5 minutes - **Servings:** 1
- 1 cup spinach
- 1 apple
- 1 cup pineapple 1tsp. of flax seeds
- ½ cup filtered water

Add all ingredients in a high-power blender and pulse until smooth. Pour the smoothie into two glasses and serve immediately.

Nutrition Facts: Calories 102kcal, Fat 0.3 g, Carbohydrate 18.5 g, Protein 1 g

482. Kale Smoothie

Preparation Time: 5 minutes - **Servings:** 1
- 1 cup kale
- ½ mango
- ½ banana
- 1 tbsp. chia seeds
- ¼ cup coconut milk, unsweetened ½ cup filtered water

Add all ingredients in a high-power blender and pulse until smooth. Pour the smoothie into two glasses and serve immediately

Nutrition Facts: Calories 156kcal, Fat 4.5 g, Carbohydrate 20.5 g, Protein 3.2 g

483. Lettuce Smoothie

Preparation Time: 5 minutes - **Servings:** 1
- ½ small head of lettuce 3 fresh plums, seeded
- ½ banana
- 1 tbsp. linseed ½ cucumber
- ½ cup almond milk, unsweetened

Add all ingredients in a high-power blender and pulse until smooth. Pour the smoothie into two glasses and serve immediately.

Nutrition Facts: Calories 138kcal, Fat 2.5 g, Carbohydrate 19.8 g, Protein 3g

484. Chocolate strawberry milk

Preparation time: 5 minutes - Cooking time: 0 minutes - Serving: 1
- 150 g strawberries, peeled and halved
- 1 tbsp cocoa powder (100 percent cocoa)
- 10 g pitted Medjool dates
- 10 g walnuts
- 200 ml milk or dairy-free alternative

Put all ingredients in a powerful mixer and stir until smooth. Once the matcha has dissolved, add the rest of the juice.
Nutrition: Carbohydrates: 16 Fat: 6 Protein: 3 Kcal: 130

485. Pineapple Lassi

Preparation time: 5 minutes - Cooking time: 0 minutes - Serving: 1
- 200 g pineapple, cut into pieces
- 150 g Greek yogurt
- 4–5 ice cubes
- 1 teaspoon ground turmeric

Put all ingredients in a powerful mixer and stir until smooth. Once the matcha has dissolved, add the rest of the juice. Just add some water and blend until you have the consistency you want, if the mixture is too thick.
Nutrition: Carbohydrates: 13 Fat: 3 Protein: 2 Kcal: 90

486. Sirt shot

Preparation time: 5 minutes - Cooking time: 0 minutes - Serving: 1
- 3–5 cm (10 g) turmeric root, peeled
- 4–6 cm (25 g) fresh ginger, peeled
- ½ medium-sized (70 g) apple, unpeeled Juice of ¼ lemon
- Pinch of black pepper

Put all ingredients in a powerful mixer and stir until smooth. Once the matcha has dissolved, add the rest of the juice. Just add some water and blend until you have the consistency you want, if the mixture is too thick.
Nutrition: Carbohydrates: 7 Fat: 10 Protein: 2 Kcal: 110

487. Hot chocolate eggnog

Preparation time: 5 minutes. - Cooking Time: 2 Minutes. - Servings: 4
- 4 cups light eggnog
- Whipped cream for topping
- 2 cups white chocolate chips
- Sprinkles for topping

Put in eggnog and white chocolate into a medium pot. Warm over low flame but do not let it achieve boiling, let it simmer till chocolate melts, one to two minutes.
Mix properly and pour drink into serving cups. In a swirling manner pour whipped cream on top and garnish using sprinkles. Have a blast!
Nutrition: Carbohydrates: 8 Fat: 3 Protein: 1 Kcal: 100

488. Mint julep

Preparation time: 5 minutes - Cooking Time: 15 Minutes - Servings: 2
- 2 tablespoon peppermint simple syrup
- 4 ½ cups cranberry ginger ale
- 4 ½ candy canes for garnish
- 4 ½ sprigs fresh pine for garnish
- 1 cup crushed ice

Distribute peppermint syrup among the bottom of four glasses.
Put in crushed ice and pour on cranberry ginger ale. Add peppermint sprigs and candy canes in all the drinks. Have a blast.
Nutrition: Calories: 160 Fat: 4.5g. Carbs: 33.7g. Protein: 1.8g. Fiber: 0g.

489. Gingerbread latte

Preparation time: 10 minutes - Cooking Time: 3 hours - Servings: 4
- 4 cups whole milk
- 3 cups brewed strong coffee
- 4 cinnamon sticks
- 1/3 cup granulated sugar
- 1/2 tsp ground allspice
- 1/4 tsp ground cloves
- 1 tsp nutmeg powder
- Whipped cream
- 2 tsp ginger powder
- Caramel sauce

Mini gingerbread sweets
Put in all ingredients excluding for topping ones in a slow cooker; Mix properly.
Cover cooker: let it cook over high setting for almost three hours or over low setting for four hours.
Distribute drink among the mugs. In a swirling manner pour whipped cream on top, and then caramel sauce.
Garnish using gingerbread sweets and Have a blast!
Nutrition: Calories: 389 Fat: 34.6g. Carbs: 20.7g. Protein: 4.8g. Fiber: 0g.

490. Chili chocolate

Preparation time: 5 minutes - Cooking time: 0 minutes - Serving: 1
- 1 chili
- 250 ml milk or non-dairy
- Alternative 1 teaspoon cocoa powder (100 percent)
- 35 g dark chocolate (70 percent cocoa solids),
- 1 teaspoon grated date syrup

Halve the chilies and cut into 6 or 7 pieces. Place the remaining ingredients in a small saucepan and bring to a boil over medium to high heat, stirring periodically, in order not to burn or boil the milk.
For 2-3 minutes, simmer gently, then remove from heat and leave to steep for 1 minute. Pass and serve through a fine sieve.
Nutrition: Carbohydrates: 17 Fat: 9 Protein: 4 Kcal: 150

491. Irish coffee

Preparation Time: 15 minutes - **Cooking Time:** 0 minutes - **Servings:** 1
- cl of cane sugar syrup (or 2 pieces of sugar)
- 2 cl of fresh cream
- 4 cl of coffee
- 3 cl of whiskey (bourbon, whiskey)

1. Make the "Irish Coffee" recipe directly in the glass.
2. Heat the whiskey with the sugar (at low heat so as not to boil the whiskey) in a saucepan stirring. Prepare a black coffee and pour it over the hot and sweet whiskey, stir slightly. Pour everything into the formerly rinsed glass with warm water and coat the surface with lightly beaten cream,

its ready! Savor without delay. To make your cream work better, place it in the freezer for 20 minutes before vigorously whipping it.

3. Despite some rumors of modern times, Irish coffee is not supposed to have the three separate floors. Other variants can be made with whipped cream instead of fresh cream, liquid cane sugar instead of powdered sugar or replace the traditional whiskey with whiskey or bourbon. Still, the original recipe is the one explained above.

4. Serve in a glass type "mug."

5. Add any grated chocolate to the cream.

Nutrition: Calories: 90 Fat: 2 g Carbohydrates: 4 g Protein: 14 g

492. Caramel coffee

Preparation Time: 15 minutes - **Cooking Time:** 0 minutes - **Servings:** 1

- 15 cl of milk
- 3 cl of caramel syrup
- 1 dash of cinnamon syrup
- 1 coffee

1. Make the recipe "Coffee Caramel."

2. Make a coffee (espresso). Heat the glass under hot water and pour the caramel syrup into the bottom of the glass. Heat the milk in another container until creamy foam and pour the warm milk gently on the syrup. Pour a few drops of cinnamon syrup and pour the coffee gently over the milk (use a spoon) until you get an extra layer...

3. Serve in a tumbler type glass.

4. Sprinkle with cinnamon powder.

Nutrition: Calories: 20 Fat: 0 g Carbohydrates: 4 g Protein: 1 g

493. Latte macchiato

Preparation Time: 15 minutes - **Cooking Time:** 0 minutes - **Servings:** 1

- Coffee
- 20 cl of milk

1. Make the recipe "Latte macchiato" directly in the glass.

2. Beat the milk (preferably whole) with a whisk in a saucepan over the heat to obtain foam on the surface (or using the steam nozzle of your espresso machine).

3. Pour warm milk into a heat-resistant glass (thick walls), blocking the foam with a spatula.

4. Add the milk foam on the hot milk.

5. Finally, gently pour a strong espresso (sweetened according to taste) on the frothed milk.

6. Since whole milk has a higher density than espresso, the latter will be placed above the milk.

7. Serve in a tumbler type glass.

8. To serve, you can fill the milk foam with chocolate flakes, liquid caramel, cocoa powder, cinnamon or other spices.

Nutrition: Calories: 80 Fat: 5 g Carbohydrates: 5 g Protein: 3 g

494. Latte Macchiato Caramel

Preparation Time: 15 minutes - **Cooking Time:** 0 minutes - **Servings:** 6

- 1 l of milk
- 20 cl of coffee
- 10 cl of caramel syrup

1. Make the recipe "Latte Macchiato Caramel" in the pan.

2. Heat the milk and prepare 20 cl of hot black coffee. Divide the milk into 4 large glasses and froth the milk with an emulsifier, electric whisk, or steam nozzle on your coffee maker until you have 2 to 3 cm of milk foam.

3. Pour about 2cl of caramel syrup into each glass and slowly pour 5cl of coffee.

4. The coffee will come just below the foam of milk, to form 3 layers: the milk at the bottom, the coffee, and the milk froth above.

5. Serve in a cup-type glass.

6. Pour a little caramel syrup over the milk foam.

Nutrition: Calories: 140 Fat: 5 g Carbohydrates: 22 g Protein: 2 g

495. Coffee Cream with Caramel Milk Foam

Preparation Time: 15 minutes - **Cooking Time:** 0 minutes - **Servings:** 4

- Grand Cru Volluto capsule (to prepare 40 ml of Espresso coffee) 100 ml of milk to prepare milk foam Teaspoon caramel syrup
- 25 ml / 5 teaspoons of cream (already prepared or homemade according to the method indicated below)
- Ingredients for the preparation of 250 ml of homemade cream:
- 250 ml semi-skimmed milk
- 2 egg yolks
- 50 g of white sugar
- Half vanilla pod cut lengthwise
- Materials
- Espresso Cup (80 Ml)
- Recipe Spoon Ritual

1. Bring the milk to a boiling point along with half a vanilla pod in a casserole dish

2. Beat the egg yolks inside a bowl with the sugar

3. Continue beating the yolks and sugar while adding the milk with the half vanilla pod

4. Then, return the mixture to the pan and allow it to thicken over low heat (do not let the mixture boil to prevent it from cutting)

5. Check the consistency of the cream with a spoon and, as soon as the cream begins to adhere to the spoon, remove the pan from the heat

6. Keep stirring the mixture to keep it soft and creamy

7. Take out the vanilla bean, scrape it with a knife to remove the seeds and put it back in the cream

8. Prepare a Volluto (25 ml) in an Espresso cup or a small Nespresso recipe glass and add 25 ml / five teaspoons of the homemade cream or ready-made cream

9. Prepare milk foam with the steam nozzle of your Nespresso machine or the Aeroccino milk frother and add the caramel syrup as soon as the foam begins to form

10. Cover the coffee cream with the caramel-flavored milk foam and serve immediately

Nutrition: Calories: 26 Fat: 1.47 g Carbohydrates: 2.91 g Protein: 0.39 g

496. Hot and Cold Vanilla Espresso with Caramel Foam and Cookies

Preparation Time: 15 minutes - **Cooking Time:** 15 minutes - **Servings:** 4

For hot and cold vanilla coffee:

- Two capsules of Grand Cru Volluto
- A scoop of vanilla ice cream
- Three tablespoons of milk foam

- Two teaspoons of caramel liquid
- For the cookies:
- 70 g softened butter
- 70 g of sugar
- Teaspoon honey
- Egg
- 100 g flour
- A pinch of salt
- 50 g grated chocolate

For hazelnut caramel:
- 50 g whole hazelnuts
- 40 g of sugar
- Two tablespoons of water

1. For hot and cold vanilla coffee:
2. Prepare the milk foam, add the liquid caramel, and reserve it
3. Prepare two coffees in a large cup and pour them into a cold glass
4. Add the vanilla ice cream ball immediately and cover it with the milk foam
5. For cookies:
6. Preheat oven to 150 ° C
7. Heat sugar and water until caramelized, remove from heat and add crushed hazelnuts
8. Place the hazelnuts on a sheet of vegetable paper and roast them in the oven for 10 min, moving them occasionally
9. Put the butter, sugar, salt, honey and egg in a large bowl
10. Beat it all for a few seconds until you get a smooth mixture
11. Add caramelized hazelnuts and grated chocolate
12. Raise the oven temperature to 180 ° C
13. Put small balls of dough on the baking sheet lined with vegetable paper and bake for about 15 min
14. Let them cool on a rack
Nutrition: Calories: 190 Fat: 11 g Carbohydrates: 150 g Protein: .27 g

497. Espresso with Cottage Cheese, Lime and Brazil Nuts

Preparation Time: 5 minutes - **Cooking Time:** 20 minutes - **Servings:** 6
- One capsule of Grand Cru Volluto or Volluto Decaffeinato
- 550 g cottage cheese
- 100 g of sugar
- The juice of a lime
- Two egg whites
- Three jelly sheets or a teaspoon of agar 80 g of Brazil nuts

1. Roast the Brazil nuts in a pan and mash them finely
2. Book them
3. Dip the jelly leaves in cold water to soften them
4. Grate and squeeze the file
5. Boil 100 ml of water with sugar and lime juice for 5 minutes
6. Remove from heat and add the drained gelatin and lime zest
7. Beat the egg whites and mount them until stiff
8. Pour three-quarters of the lime syrup over the egg whites without stopping to beat and then add the cottage cheese to the mixture
9. Divide the crushed nuts into the six molds and cover them using a cottage cheese mousse
10. Pour the remaining lime syrup over and put the molds in the refrigerator for 4 hours

11. Serve it with a Grand Cru Volluto
Nutrition: Calories: 183 Fat: 5.31 g Carbohydrates: 5.5 g Protein: 27 g

498. Coffee with Malice

Preparation Time: 5 minutes - **Cooking Time:** 5 minutes - **Servings:** 4
- One intense espresso coffee sachet
- 1 splash whiskey
- 1 splash whole milk or cream

1. You can use the dolce gusto machine, but if you don't have one, you can do it with a good quality soluble coffee loaded. All right; Put the coffee sachet in the coffee maker and select the amount of water to pour.
2. Activate the hot water until it stops. Have whiskey on hand.
3. Pour a little squirt of whiskey, heat a little cream or milk, and add it to coffee.
4. Ready, you can add sugar or sweetener if it's your taste. I prefer it as it is. With its bitter touch.
Nutrition: Calories: 394 Fat: 9 g Carbohydrates: 67 g Protein: 10 g

499. Viennese coffee

Preparation Time: 5 minutes - **Cooking Time:** 0 minutes - **Servings:** 1
- Espresso coffee to your liking.
- Whole milk (if you are in full operation bikini... skimmed)
- White sugar
- Whipped cream
- Shavings chocolate

1. Take the coffee capsule. You put it in the machine and let it do its job.
2. You fill the glass of milk, add your healthy dose of sugar, and stir.
3. Decorate with a good tuft of cream and chocolate chips.
4. As you can see, very, very difficult to do. Having just spent the day.
Nutrition: Calories: 251 Fat: 27 g Carbohydrates: 0.63 g Protein: 0.62 g

500. Coffee mousse

Preparation Time: 5 minutes - **Cooking Time:** 0 minutes - **Servings:** 6
- 4 sheets jelly
- 125 ml of espresso coffee
- 2 tablespoons. Baileys
- 100 gr. sugar
- Two egg whites
- 200 ml 35% mg whipping cream

1. We put into hydrating the gelatin.
2. We prepare a coffee.
3. We ride the egg whites with the sugar about to snow.
4. We semi-cream.
5. Melt the jello in the hot coffee and add the Baileys.
6. Add the coffee to tablespoons to the whites mounted.
7. Add the whipped cream.
8. We pour the mixture into 6 glasses that we can decorate with sprinkled cocoa powder. In my case, I prepared a coffee jelly.
9. Let cool inside the fridge for a few hours and go!
Nutrition: Calories: 2 Fat: 0.5 g Carbohydrates: 4 g Protein: 0.28 g

The Sirtfood Diet Three-Week Meal Plan

Week One

Day 1
Breakfast: Mushroom Tacos
Lunch: Vegan Chili
Dinner: Chow Mein

Day 2
Breakfast: Cilantro Chili Burgers
Lunch: Vegetable Masala
Dinner: Pesto Avocado

Day 3

Breakfast: Country Chicken Breasts
Lunch: Turkey Satay Skewers
Dinner: Fried Cauliflower Rice

Day 4
Breakfast: Lamb, Butternut Squash and Date Tagine
Lunch: Miso-Marinated Baked Cod with Stir-Fried Greens and Sesame
Dinner: Celery Juice

Day 5
Breakfast: Horseradish Flaked Salmon Fillet & Kale
Lunch: Chocolate Fondue
Dinner: Chili Con Carne

Day 6
Breakfast: Chicken with Kale and Chili Salsa
Lunch: Fragrant Asian Hotpot
Dinner: Strawberry Buckwheat Tabbouleh

Day 7
Breakfast: Tomato Frittata
Lunch: Soba in a miso broth with tofu, celery, and kale
Dinner: Broccoli and Kale Green Soup

Week Two

Day 8
Breakfast: Buckwheat tabbouleh with Strawberries
Lunch: Tuscan Stewed Beans
Dinner: Indulgent Yoghurt

Day 9
Breakfast: Sirtfood Diet Chicken Breakfast Salad

Lunch: Prawn Pasta
Dinner: Lemon Salmon

Day 10
Breakfast: Buckwheat Tuna
Lunch: Asian King Prawn Stir Fry with Buckwheat Noodles
Dinner: Sirt Muesli

Day 11
Breakfast: Smoked Salmon Omelet
Lunch: Potato and Chickpea Bake
Dinner: Sweet Pepper Mix

Day 12
Breakfast: Apple and Blackcurrant Pancakes
Lunch: Kale Dhal with Buckwheat
Dinner: Tofu Curry

Day 13
Breakfast: Breakfast Shakshuka
Lunch: Cod Fish with Turmeric
Dinner: Greek Salad on a Stick

Day 14
Breakfast: Moroccan Eggs
Lunch: Grilled Salmon
Dinner: Buckwheat Chicken Noodles

Week Three

Day 15
Breakfast: Fruit and Yoghurt Muesli
Lunch: Lemon and Garlic Chili Chicken
Dinner: Smoked Salmon Super Salad

Day 16

Breakfast: Buckwheat Pancakes with Dark Chocolate Sauce
Lunch: Rocket Caesar Salad with Flax Seeds
Dinner: Turmeric Chicken and Kale Bowl

Day 17

Breakfast: Banana and Blueberry Oat Pancakes
Lunch: Vegetable Chili
Dinner: Buckwheat Chicken Noodles

Day 18
Breakfast: Turmeric Pancakes with Lemon Yoghurt
Lunch: Lemon Splash Tofu

Dinner: Sesame Chicken Salad

Day 19
Breakfast: Buckwheat Pancakes with Pineapple
Lunch: Veggie Stuffed Peppers
Dinner: Waldorf Salad

Day 20
Breakfast: Egg Whites and Pepper Omelet
Lunch: Broccoli and Turmeric Cream Soup
Dinner: Sirtfood Coleslaw

Day 21
Breakfast: Good Morning Eggs
Lunch: Chicken Salad with Sprouts
Dinner: Lemon Salmon

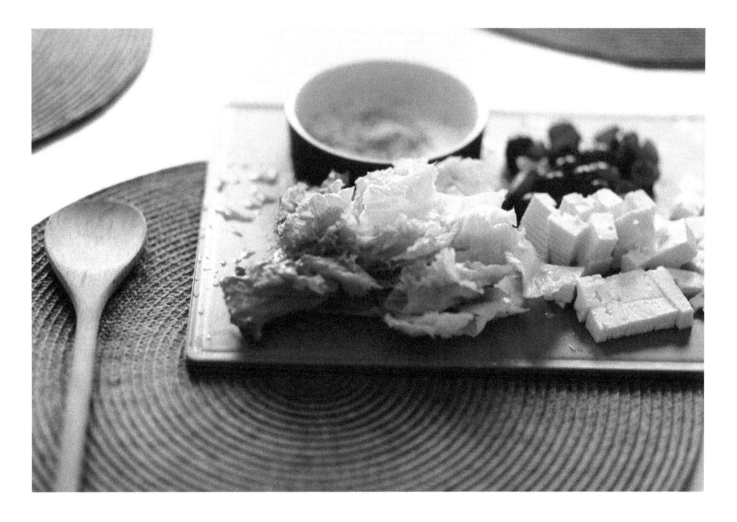

Lightning Source UK Ltd.
Milton Keynes UK
UKHW050924180321
380564UK00004B/24